Y0-BZY-891

ATLAS OF
PEDIATRIC SURGERY

Keith W. Ashcraft, M.D.

The Children's Mercy Hospital
2401 Gilham Road
Kansas City, MO 64108

W.B. SAUNDERS COMPANY
A Division of Harcourt Brace & Company
Philadelphia ■ London ■ Toronto ■ Montreal ■ Sydney ■ Tokyo

W.B. SAUNDERS COMPANY
A Division of
Harcourt Brace & Company

The Curtis Center
Independence Square West
Philadelphia, Pennsylvania 19106

Library of Congress Cataloging-in-Publication Data

Ashcraft, Keith W.

Atlas of pediatric surgery / Keith W. Ashcraft.

p.   cm.

ISBN 0–7216–3720–5

1. Children—Surgery—Atlases.   I. Title. [DNLM: 1. Surgery,
   Operative—in infancy & childhood—atlases.
   WO 517 A823a 1994]

RD137.3.A84 1994

617.9′8—dc20

DNLM/DLC   93–1848

Atlas of Pediatric Surgery   ISBN 0–7216–3720–5

Copyright © 1994 by W.B. Saunders Company

All rights reserved.   No part of this publication may be reproduced or transmitted in any form or
by any means, electronic or mechanical, including photocopy, recording, or any information stor-
age and retrieval system, without permission in writing from the publisher.

Printed in the United States of America

Last digit is the print number: 9   8   7   6   5   4   3   2   1

I would like to dedicate this atlas to Tom Holder. I first became acquainted with Tom in 1961 when I was a medical student and he was the fresh young Chief of Surgery at Children's Mercy. After spending time on the wards and especially in the operating room as a junior clerk, I knew that pediatric surgery was my logical career choice. Tom Holder provided the inspiration for this atlas and more work on it than he will admit. No matter what it says on the spine, I think everybody will recognize this as a Holder/Ashcraft product—I certainly do.

PREFACE

This atlas is a collection of surgical procedures performed in children. Some procedures are common, and some are not. They were selected for inclusion because they are procedures that will occupy much of the pediatric surgeon's operative time or because they involve principles that carry over to many surgical procedures that are not described.

I learned most of what I know about surgical technique from Tom Holder, who brought the concepts and skills taught him by Robert Gross to Kansas City at a time when I had just happened on the scene. Other surgeons and residents have taught me many things, some of which have shaped the way I approach a procedure. Robert Gross produced an atlas in 1970, and in the preface to that atlas he expressed as well as can be expressed two concepts to which I thoroughly ascribe:

1. If an operation is difficult, you are not doing it properly.
2. There are, and always will be, operations that are not "routine" and which must be done as individualized undertakings, depending upon the variable pathology and conditions found at the time and the various ways in which different surgeons handle them. Aside from these, there are a tremendous number of operations which can be "regularized" and can be performed by using standardized, repeatable techniques; this means essentially that the same sequential technical steps are used every time that operation is performed. This does not reduce the surgeon to an automaton or a grinding drudge; instead, it makes his work of better quality. Standardization implies that the operator knows exactly what he is doing and what the progressive procedure will be; it also makes him work expeditiously. Furthermore, teamwork is improved because each member of the group knows what is going to be done next; the assistant is familiar with the precise step which is to follow, and the scrub nurse anticipates and provides the exact instrument or suture which will be used next. The whole operation clicks along in a quiet, rapid, and orderly fashion. It is highly pleasant to work in this manner, and it safely reduces the length of operating time and anesthesia, which are obvious benefits for the patient. In commonly performed operations, there is no excuse for diddling around; these operations should be technical jobs which are thought out ahead of time, can be practiced, and can be carried out with maximum order and dispatch. The whole team moves with smoothness of action, maintenance of quiet atmosphere, and attainment of a high degree of surgical skill, all of which are most worthy objectives.[1]

Constructing a surgical procedure that can be carried out in a logical and smooth progression and with little wasted motion establishes self-confidence. Agonizing over any operative procedure, particularly those that are low risk and done in virgin territory, prevents self-confidence. The belief that you, the reader, are the proper surgeon for the job must be developed through careful thought and planning so that it looks easy to those who are helping you.

This atlas will appeal most to residents who are in the process of forming their own style and technique. Take from it what you wish and discard the rest. Our techniques are not the only way to do each procedure, but they do work.

Leave your patient looking as nice as possible. Scars that do not follow body lines are ugly. Skin sutures and staples leave ugly marks that say to the patient, "I didn't care enough about you to do a subcuticular closure." Most parents will feel that if you leave their child with a minimal scar, you probably did the same sort of careful work on the inside. I think so, too!

Finally, I want to thank W.B. Saunders and our artist Drew Strawbridge. Both put up with many revisions. This book was largely produced through the effort of my secretary, Dena Ramsey, to whom I owe a debt of gratitude.

Reference

1. Gross RE: An Atlas of Children's Surgery. Philadelphia, WB Saunders, 1970.

CONTENTS

1 Incisions 1

2 Dermoids 5

3 Preauricular Sinus 7

4 Branchial Cleft Sinus 11

5 Thyroglossal Duct/Cyst 13

6 Tracheostomy 17

7 Vascular Access 21

8 Minithoracotomy for Empyema 26

9 Pectus Repair 29

10 Esophageal Atresia/Tracheoesophageal Fistula 37

11 Mediastinal Lesions 45

12 Colon Interposition 49

13   Reversed Gastric Tube **57**

14   Congenital Diaphragmatic Hernia **61**

15   Fundoplication **67**

16   Achalasia **75**

17   Stamm Gastrostomy **79**

18   Pyloromyotomy **85**

19   Duodenal Obstruction **91**

20   Malrotation **97**

21   Portoenterostomy (Kasai Procedure) **103**

22   Choledochal Cyst **111**

23   Splenectomy **117**

24   Subtotal and Total Pancreatectomy **121**

25   Splenorenal Shunt **127**

26   Mesocaval and Portocaval Shunt **133**

27   Intestinal Atresia **139**

28   Meconium Ileus **149**

29   Necrotizing Enterocolitis **155**

30   Intussusception **161**

31   Intestinal Duplication **165**

32 Meckel's Diverticulum **169**

33 Colostomy **173**

34 Omphalocele and Gastroschisis **179**

35 Mini-Pena Procedure **185**

36 Pena Procedure **189**

37 Soave Pull-through **199**

38 Duhamel Procedure **205**

39 Rectal Prolapse **215**

40 Sacrococcygeal Teratoma **219**

41 Presacral Teratoma **225**

42 Fistula-in-ano **229**

43 Endorectal Pull-through **233**

44 Cloaca **239**

45 Inguinal Hernia **249**

46 Umbilical Hernia **263**

47 Orchiopexy **267**

48 Wilms' Tumor **277**

49 The Acute Scrotum **285**

50 Duckett Urethroplasty **291**

51 MAGPI Urethroplasty **301**

52 Adrenogenital Syndrome **305**

Index **315**

CHAPTER

1

Incisions

The prime consideration when making a surgical incision is to provide exposure for visualization and access for the operative procedure. Given a choice of incisions, the one that provides the best cosmetic result should be chosen. In general, those incisions that follow the lines of Langhorn provide the best aesthetic results. Those incisions that are made at right angles to a natural fold tend to create more obvious scars. Incisions that cross joint folds at right angles should be avoided.

The younger the child, the more elastic and mobile are the skin and subcutaneous tissue—a factor that allows more leeway in the selection of the skin incision. A chest incision in girls should be planned in such a way as to avoid disfiguring the developing breast.

Examples of incisions in different areas of the body are depicted in Figures 1A through 1C.

Scars resulting from an operation will be carried throughout life. The eventual cosmetic result ultimately depends more on the degree of scarring than on the position of the incision. Meticulous technique—avoiding tension on the skin and avoiding skin sutures—tends to give a more satisfactory scar. Subcuticular wound closure using Steri-Strips yields the most cosmetically pleasing result.

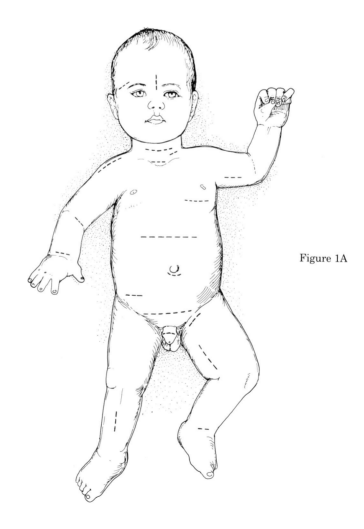

Figure 1A

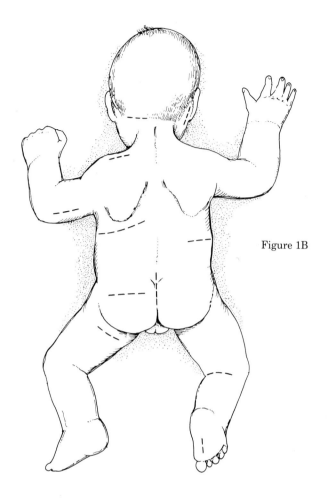

Figure 1B

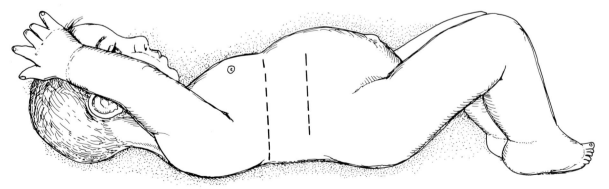

Figure 1C

CHAPTER

2

Dermoids

Dermoids are commonly seen in children. They are most often at the lateral aspect of the eyebrow on either side (Fig. 2), followed by the occipital region and the midline of the neck just above the sternal notch. Dermoids may best be thought of as a skin cyst entrapped (skin side inside) without connection to the surface. The desquamated skin accumulates within and produces the smegma-like content of the dermoid. Although we have not seen infections in dermoid cysts, they have been reported. Dermoids are unsightly, and because of their gradual enlargement over time, they need to be removed.

It is important not to shave the hair of the eyebrow, because it may not grow back. An incision is made either in the eyebrow through the hair or just above it, overlying the dermoid cyst. Dermoids should be approached sharply and with caution. They are best removed intact, ensuring that all of the cyst wall has been removed.

Dermoids located over the side of the skull sometimes have a communication through the skull, resulting in a dumbbell-shaped portion of dermoid within the cranial cavity. These are detected by skull radiographs, which show a small hole directly underlying the superficial dermoid. These patients should be referred to a neurosurgeon.

Dermoids have a surprisingly good blood supply. In spite of careful hemostasis with electrocautery, an ecchymosis may develop in the region, producing a black eye. Subcuticular skin closure and Steri-Strips are preferred to minimize the scarring.

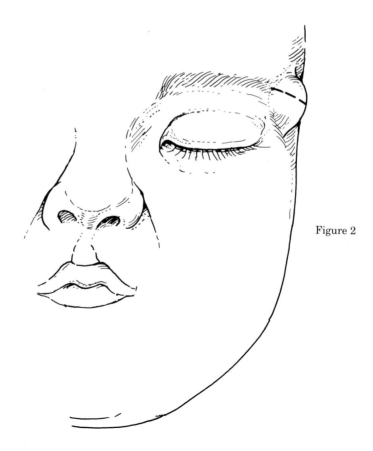

Figure 2

3

Preauricular sinus

Excision of a preauricular cyst or sinus should be performed when there is no active infection. Infection may require incision, drainage, or treatment with antibiotics until all the inflammation has subsided. Lesions that have been previously infected present greater vascularity and scarring problems than those that have not.

An elliptical incision is made around the skin opening in the natural fold in front of the helix (Fig. 3A), extending down, if necessary, in front of the tragus. The tract tends to extend inferiorly. There may be attachments to the cartilage of the tragus or to that of the external auditory canal. All remnants of the tract must be removed (Fig. 3B) (including shaving of the adjacent cartilage), or a recurrence is likely. In patients who have had a previous infection, particular care should be exercised to avoid injury to the temporal zygomatic branch of the facial nerve; such injury is more likely because of the increased vascularity, which may obscure visibility, and the fibrous reaction, which may alter the anatomy. The subcutaneous tissues are approximated and the skin is closed with interrupted subcuticular sutures of absorbable material. Collodion or Steri-Strips are then applied.

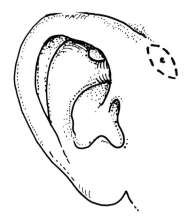

Figure 3A

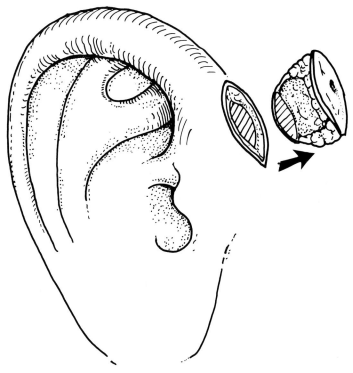

Figure 3B

Branchial cleft sinus

A complete branchial cleft sinus is more common than either a remnant or an isolated cyst. Sinuses at the second cleft are the most common and extend from the anterior border of the sternomastoid to the pharynx by way of the carotid bifurcation.

The patient is placed under general endotracheal anesthesia with the neck extended by using a rolled towel placed beneath the shoulders. The head is turned to the opposite side. The skin of the entire neck is prepped and draped up to the level of the mandible. A small 4–0 or 5–0 blue or black monofilament suture is pushed as far as possible into the tract to aid the dissection. As an alternative, a small amount of methylene blue can be injected into the punctum.

A transverse elliptical (1 to 1.5 cm) incision is made around the punctum of the sinus, which is along the anterior border of the sternomastoid muscle (Fig. 4). A mosquito forceps may be used to grasp the orifice and hold the suture/stent in place. Dissection is facilitated by retracting the wound superiorly and applying gentle traction on the sinus tract. The dissection proceeds superiorly and medially, staying close to the tract. The tract turns medially to join the pharynx inferior to the hypoglossal nerve and between the internal and external carotid arteries. If the sinus is a relatively short one (2 or 3 cm), it can be removed through a single incision. For longer tracts, a counterincision is made along the anterior border of the upper third of the sternomastoid. The two incisions are joined subcutaneously, allowing the distal sinus tract to be passed upward and brought out through the upper incision. The sinus is dissected, through the second incision, to its junction with the pharynx. The sinus tract is then suture ligated using absorbable suture material at the pharyngeal junction. Bleeding is usually not a problem, but hemostasis must be meticulously controlled. The skin incisions are closed with subcuticular sutures. A soft rubber drain may be left for 24 hours.

Hematoma is the most frequent complication.

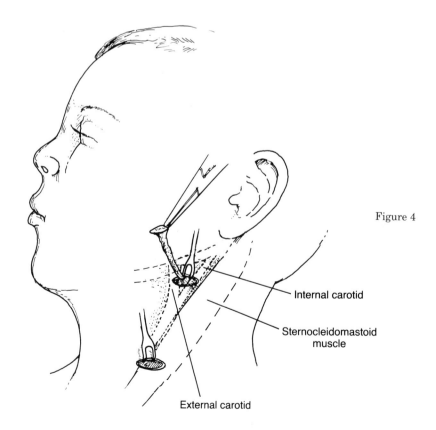

Figure 4

Internal carotid

Sternocleidomastoid muscle

External carotid

5

Thyroglossal duct/cyst

Any midline cyst above the level of the thyroid must be suspected to be a thyroglossal duct/cyst. Virtually always there is a duct connecting the cyst to the foramen cecum at the base of the tongue. These lesions contain viscous "saliva" and are much easier to remove before infection than after. The presence of such a lesion is sufficient indication for surgical excision.

The operation is done under general endotracheal anesthesia. The neck is extended by placing a rolled towel under the shoulders, and a transverse incision is made at the level of the hyoid bone rather than over the mass (Fig. 5A). This provides exposure for the dissection of the suprahyoid duct and places the scar more in the submandibular area than on the neck. The incision is deepened through the platysma to expose the cyst, which is dissected up to the hyoid bone. The muscles attaching above and below the hyoid bone are divided with electrocautery at their insertion into the hyoid. The mid portion of the hyoid bone is freed so that about 1 to 1.5 cm of the hyoid may be removed with the specimen (Fig. 5B). The bone is then divided laterally with small bone cutters.

The dissection continues upward into the base of the tongue. The endotracheal tube within the pharynx is easily palpable. The duct is suture ligated near the base of the tongue with absorbable suture material, and hemostasis is meticulously controlled with electrocautery (Fig. 5C). A small, soft rubber drain is left deep to the hyoid. The deep muscles are approximated, and the platysma is closed with continuous absorbable sutures. The drain is brought out through the mid portion of the incision, and the skin is closed with running subcuticular sutures.

The drain is removed the first postoperative day.

The most serious complication of this operation is a postoperative hematoma, which may cause airway obstruction.

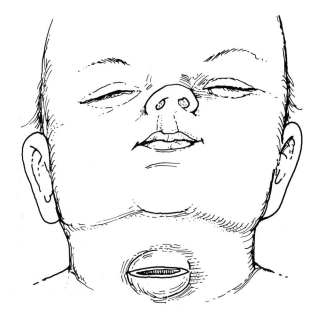

Figure 5A

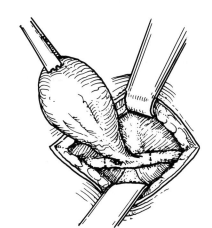

Figure 5B

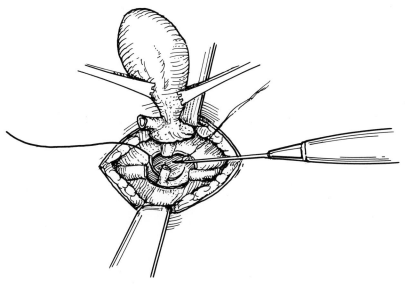

Figure 5C

6

Tracheostomy

It has long been said that the indication for tracheostomy was to have thought of it. Actually, the indication for performing a tracheostomy in a pediatric patient is to facilitate repair or healing of a laryngeal lesion, to provide an airway while a patient with an obstructive lesion grows, and to enable a patient who is in need of long-term ventilation to eat while also being intubated. A tracheostomy is not innocuous.

Tracheotomy in infants should be done in the operating room with the infant under general endotracheal anesthesia. The patient is positioned with the neck extended as far as possible by a roll placed under the shoulders (Fig. 6A). A transverse skin incision is in a skin fold about 1 cm above the sternal notch. The incision is carried through the skin, subcutaneous tissue, and platysma down to the strap muscles, which are separated in the midline. The isthmus of the thyroid is then retracted superiorly. The anterior aspect of the trachea is exposed, but extensive skeletal muscle dissection should be avoided. Traction sutures are then placed around about the third tracheal ring, avoiding the cricoid and first ring (Fig. 6B). A vertical incision is then made through two or three rings and should be of sufficient size to allow the introduction of an appropriately sized tracheotomy tube.

Depending on its size, the skin incision may be left open, or a single suture may be placed on either side of the tracheotomy; approximating the platysma and subcutaneous tissue may be helpful. The tube should be tied snugly in place with a knot that will not slip. The tracheostomy tape ends are cut short to prevent someone loosening the tie (Fig. 6C). In a small child, the position of the tube is critical. Before leaving the operating room, the patency of the airway should be determined with the patient's head in various positions. The traction sutures are left long and tied, marked "left" and "right," and taped to the chest (Fig. 6D). If the tracheotomy tube becomes displaced within the first few postoperative days, these sutures will be extremely helpful in repositioning it. Currently the tracheotomy tube most widely used in infants and small children is the Shiley plastic tube with a 15-mm anesthetic fitting.

The most serious complications of tracheostomy are dislodgement, erosion into the innominate artery, and misplacement through the first ring or the cricoid. Good exposure is mandatory, and the procedure requires an experienced surgeon.

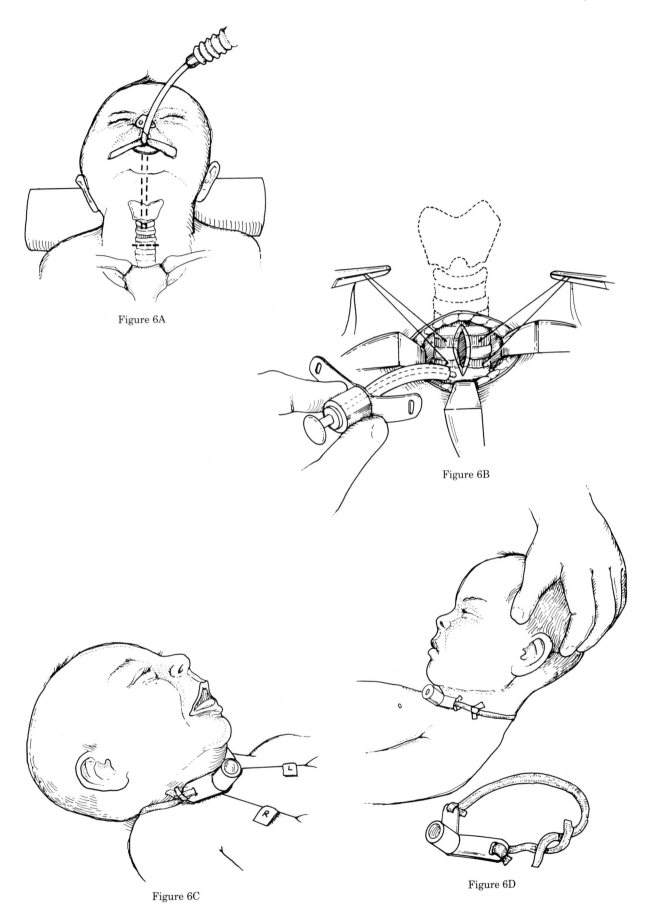

Figure 6A

Figure 6B

Figure 6C

Figure 6D

CHAPTER

7

Vascular access

Vascular access is necessary in pediatric patients for administration of anesthesia, for postoperative care, and for administration of medications. Many devices are available, the most common being the plastic catheter-over-needle, used most often for peripheral vascular access.

The most common superficial peripheral vein is the greater saphenous vein at the ankle (7A). This vein is used in patients who will not be expected to ambulate before the need for vascular access is complete. The best way to approach this vein is to place a tourniquet slightly below the knee; this produces distention of the vein. Bright light is preferred to allow "visualization" of the vein through the skin, if possible. However, palpation, along with the knowledge that the vein is almost universally present, is the best tool for locating it. The foot is extended and either held by an assistant or placed on a padded board. We prefer to hold the foot extended with the left hand, placing the needle with the right and having an assistant thread the catheter over the needle into the vein once the blood has flashed back into the needle hub. The needle is placed through the skin with the bevel up, after first nicking the skin with the needle tip to make the opening larger than the Teflon catheter. The catheter is also loosened before insertion to make sure that it slides freely off the needle. Once the needle tip pierces the vein and blood is returned, the needle is rotated 180 degrees so that the bevel is down and the cannula will slip off the needle into the vein. When this maneuver is performed smoothly, vascular access is almost always successful.

There are times when the vessel cannot be seen or palpated. From a stab incision just below and anterior to the medial malleolus, a gentle, "fan-like" probing of the subcutaneous tissues can be done with the needle, and often the vein will be encountered. We do not advocate impaling a vessel and then withdrawing into the lumen; instead, insertion should progress very slowly so that, at first contact with the lumen of the vein, blood is returned. Rotation of the needle and advancement of the catheter are then possible.

Multiple puncture attempts with the same needle sometimes result in a small piece of fat lodging in the lumen, and flashback of blood is thus prevented. The needle may be irrigated to ensure patency.

The veins of the back of the hand are the next best site for vascular access in infants and children (Fig. 7B). Although these are not as constant, there are usually two, either one of which may be used for access. A similar three-handed insertion technique is advocated.

On the volar surface of the hand, there is a very small unnamed vein that is almost always constant (Fig. 7E). Many anesthesiologists prefer to use this vein, even though it will accept only a small plastic catheter. It is usually quite sufficient for short-term perioperative use.

The femoral vessels represent another site that is not desirable but is available for short-term intraoperative use. The femoral artery, which usually is easily palpated, is located lateral to the femoral vein (Fig. 7F). Long-term vascular access at this site is usually impractical in children who wear diapers unless postoperative bladder decompression using a Foley catheter is part of the procedure.

Long-term vascular access for total parenteral nutrition or chemotherapy is usually accomplished through the neck or the subclavian vessels (Fig. 7C). Single-, double-, and even triple-lumen sets are available for this purpose. Access to the vein is determined by needle puncture. A guide wire is then passed to ensure that the central venous system has been reached, and the indwelling catheter is then passed over the guide wire. Sometimes this is done under fluoroscopic control, but often it is quite easily accomplished on the ward or in the operating room without fluoroscopy. The patient should be positioned so that the head is down to both distend the veins and prevent an air embolus. The skin of the neck or upper chest is prepped and draped for

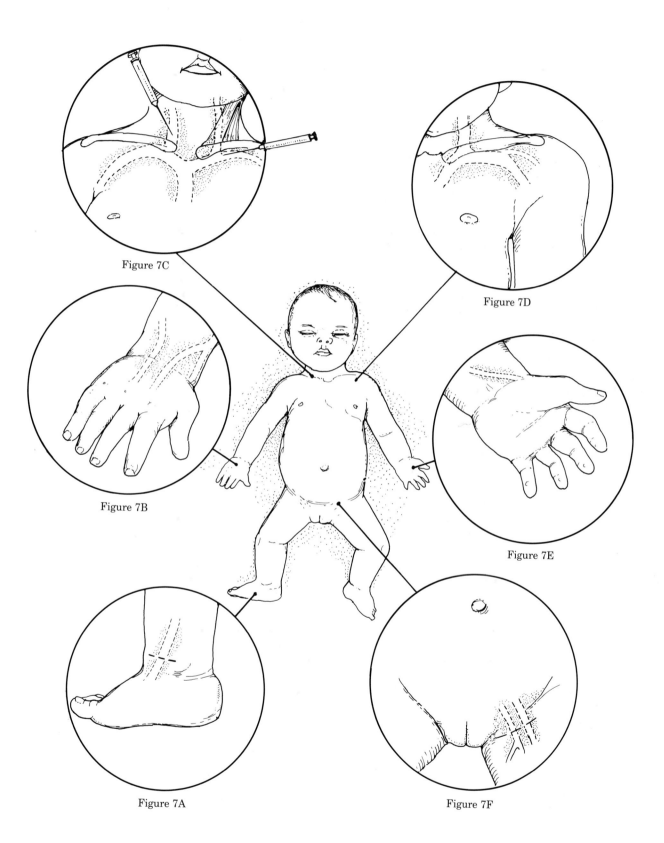

Figure 7C

Figure 7D

Figure 7B

Figure 7E

Figure 7A

Figure 7F

this sterile procedure. Gloves are used to allow handling of the catheter, which may remain in the vascular system for a period of days or weeks. Puncture of the subclavian vein at the bend in the clavicle is usually accomplished with an 18- or 20-gauge needle. Once free flow of blood has been determined, the needle is left in place, the syringe detached, and the guide wire inserted. Some guide wires are straight, whereas others have a flexible "J" tip that aids in achieving access to the superior vena cava. An electrocardiogram, if available, will often show ectopic beats once the wire reaches the atrium. The guide wire is withdrawn until the ectopy disappears. The needle is removed from the vein and taken off the guide wire, and the intravenous catheter device is then inserted over the guide wire. Before insertion, care is taken to ensure that the guide wire is longer than the venous catheter, so that if the guide wire is pushed in ahead of the catheter, it will not be lost to retrieval. Once the catheter is positioned, it is either sutured in place or held in place with a large plastic adhesive dressing (e.g., Op-Site).

Another vein used for cutdown access to the upper venous system is the cephalic vein at the deltopectoral groove (Fig. 7D). This is often used for placement of transvenous electrodes for cardiac pacing.

Cutdown may be accomplished at any of these sites depending on whether percutaneous techniques are successful. Knowledge of anatomy is most important. Cutdown on the saphenous vein at the ankle is the surest method of achieving venous access. Although percutaneous puncture of antecubital vessels in the child is not often performed, this is another potential site for cutdown. Cutdown may be necessary in the patient who has multiple injuries or is in shock and in whom the vascular system is in collapse. Under these conditions, venous distention and percutaneous puncture are unlikely.

Depending on the status of the patient, local anesthesia is generally used. Sterile technique is important except in the most dire circumstances. The skin incision should be made and blunt dissection with a fine-tipped hemostat used to locate the vein. The vein is isolated and surrounded with two ligatures. We prefer 4–0 silk if it is available, but chromic or other absorbable material may also be used. The distal vein is usually tied off. A cut into the vein allows access of a cutdown catheter; otherwise, puncture of the vein may be accomplished by a catheter-over-needle apparatus. The vein is ligated over the indwelling needle catheter.

CHAPTER

8

Minithoracotomy for empyema

Empyema often occurs in pediatric patients after staphylococcal and *Haemophilus influenzae* pneumonitis with transudation of bacteria into the pleural space. What is often a very thin fluid early becomes coagulated quickly and will form loculations that cannot be drained by thoracentesis. Placement of a chest tube into the pleural space also will not drain this gelatinous fibrinous material, and thus a small anterior thoracotomy with active suction of the fibrin from the surface of the lung and the inside of the parietal pleura is necessary. We prefer to use a submammary incision well away from the breast so that as the breast develops in girls, it will not be distorted by scar (Fig. 8). An intercostal incision approximately 2 cm long is made, and a small rib spreader inserted. Either a tonsil sucker or the open end of the plastic surgical suction tubing can be used to evacuate the gelatinous material from the inside of the chest. This tube is passed upward rather blindly and works as an effective vacuum to clean the pleural space. A chest tube is then inserted through the same incision or through a separate stab incision and left in place to drain the reactive fluid that follows the minithoracotomy. The chest tube can be removed the following day or left in place as long as drainage continues.

This procedure can be managed as well by thoracoscopy.

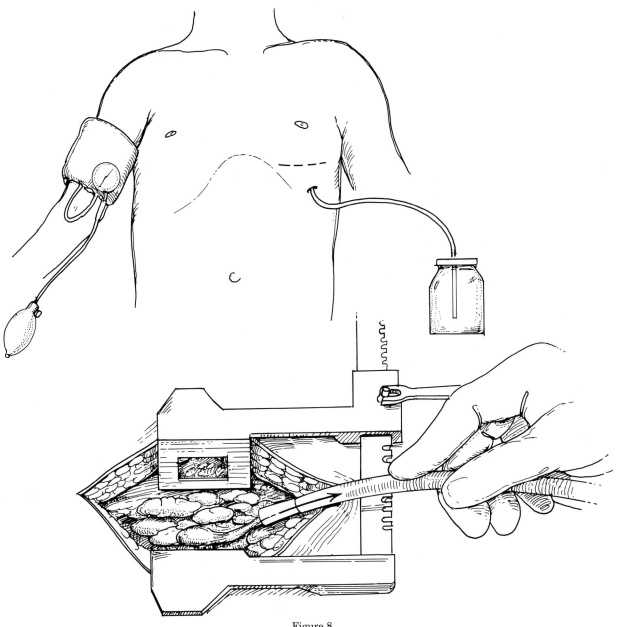

Figure 8

CHAPTER

9

Pectus repair

Repair of a pectus excavatum was formerly considered a cosmetic procedure, but repeated demonstrations that pectus deformities interfere with pulmonary function have led to the acceptance of this procedure as physiologically necessary.

The preferred age at correction is between 2½ and 4 years. A pectus deformity present at this age will not improve without operation. The procedure is well tolerated at this age, and the need for blood transfusion is reduced when compared with the same procedure performed in teenage patients. The chest capacity is improved so that as the lungs undergo final development, there is as much room for them as possible. The pectus repair, in our experience, is maintained throughout the growth spurt in 96% of patients when performed at this age.

The deformity appears to be primarily related to the inwardly curved costal cartilages, which depress the sternum and may turn the sternal ends of the ribs inward. It most commonly involves the lower costal cartilages, extending up at times to involve the second and third costal cartilages. The sternum is pushed inward, probably as a result of the force exerted by the costal cartilages rather than by internal traction. A symmetric pectus deformity usually yields the most cosmetically satisfactory repair; the asymmetric forms usually result in an asymmetric repair. We prefer a procedure, modified from that of Welch,* that utilizes no internal or external strutting.

Either a bilateral submammary incision or a vertical midline incision may be used (Figs. 9A, 9B). The vertical incision is used when the deformity extends to the second or third ribs; the submammary incision is more cosmetic, particularly in girls.

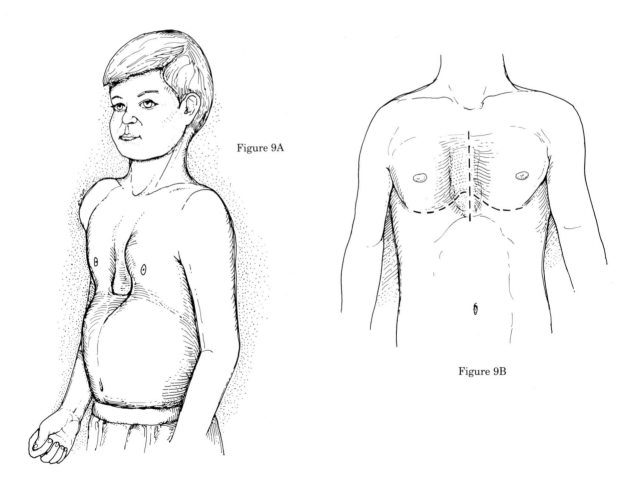

Figure 9A

Figure 9B

In both procedures, the initial incision is carried through the pectoral muscles to the level of the sternum and the ribs, and myocutaneous flaps are developed superiorly, inferiorly, and laterally to expose the sternum and all of the deformed costal cartilages (Fig. 9C). Generous use of the electrocautery and, more recently, the argon beam coagulator will minimize blood loss. The sternum is exposed to the interspace above the most superiorly deformed costal cartilage; its anterior table will be "wedged" out at this level.

Beginning superiorly, the perichondrium of the deformed costal cartilage is incised as nearly as possible directly over its center and along its length from the end of the rib to its junction with the sternum or manubrium. Vertical extensions at the extremities of this perichondrial incision allow the perichondrium to be lifted bluntly off the rib and turned upward and downward so that the cartilage can be dissected from the perichondrium posteriorly. The cartilage should be lifted by a blunt periosteal elevator passed beneath it, transected, and removed to its junction with the rib laterally and to its junction with the manubrium medially. The easiest way to do this is to have the surgeon dissect the ribs on the side opposite his or her location, with the assistant holding a retractor for lifting the myocutaneous flaps for exposure. For the second side, the roles are reversed. It is easiest to dissect the perichondrium off the costal cartilages closer to the sternum than farther away. Once the proper plane is found, the "whale tail" blunt periosteal elevator is used to strip the perichondrium from the entire length of cartilage. The lower cartilages often have bridges to the next lower cartilage, which makes the dissection more difficult. The perichondrium should be incised with the electrocautery across these bridges and turned back so that the bridge can be divided sharply and each deformed costal cartilage removed completely.

Usually the lowest costal cartilage that must be totally removed is the one that attaches to the sternum. The deformed tips of the floating ribs rarely cause any problem, although flaring of the lower chest may be extensive in some of these deformities.

---

*Shamberger RC, Welch KJ: Chest wall deformities. In Ashcraft KW, Holder TM, eds: Pediatric Surgery. 2nd ed. Philadelphia, WB Saunders, 1993, p 146.

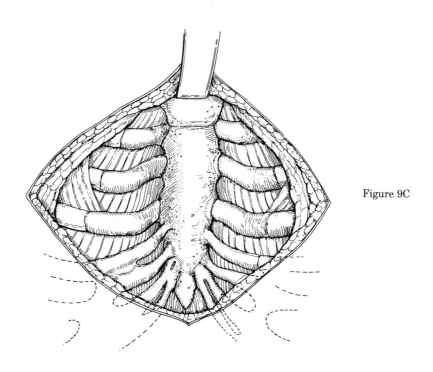

Figure 9C

The xiphoid is removed (Fig. 9*D*). The resultant longitudinal defect in the rectus sheath later will be closed transversely to help support the lower end of the sternum in a forward position.

The sternum and manubrium in the interspace just above the most superiorly excised costal cartilage is then cut with an osteotome, taking a wedge out of the anterior table (Fig. 9*E*). A finger inserted behind the sternum allows the posterior table to be broken. The sternum is thus hinged and brought forward at the point of its osteotomy. Cutting only the anterior table eliminates the need for sutures to support the osteotomy. At this point, all of the bent costal cartilages that were pushing the sternum posteriorly have been removed, and the sternum should be free enough that expansion of the lungs and the pressure of the heart will push it forward.

The defect left by excision of the xiphoid is then closed in a horizontal fashion with several permanent interrupted sutures, thus shortening fascial attachments of the rectus to the sternum, which helps to hold the sternum forward (Fig. 9*E*).

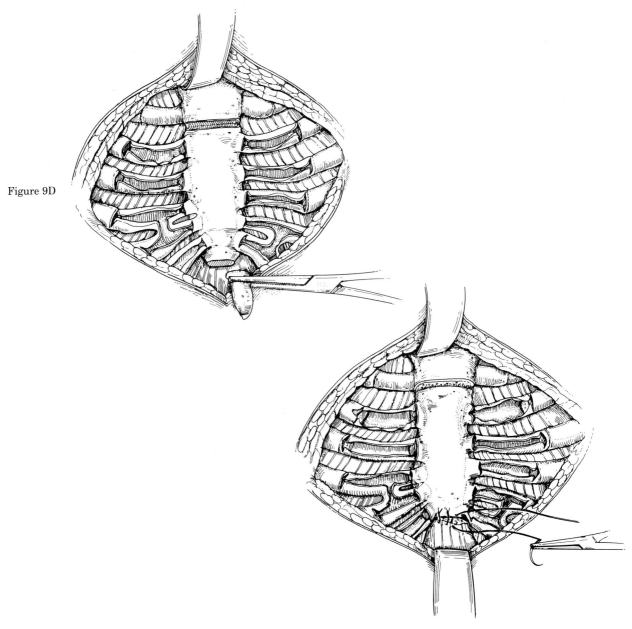

Figure 9D

Figure 9E

Reefing of the perichondrium is then begun, using permanent interrupted 2–0 silk sutures placed in a figure-of-8 manner. Reefing is accomplished posteriorly in the perichondria starting with the highest rib by placing one suture posteriorly and then reapproximating the anterior cut edges of the perichondrium anteriorly with another suture (Figs. 9*F* through 9*H*). The perichondrium is reefed on the right side by placing one suture posteriorly and one suture anteriorly and then crossing over and reefing the perichondrium on the left side, again with one suture posteriorly and one anteriorly. The next rib is reefed with one suture posteriorly and two anteriorly. The third is reefed with two sutures posteriorly and two anteriorly. It is important to alternate from one side to the other so that the sternum is not deflected either to the right or to the left, as might occur if one side was reefed completely before the other side.

An impressive amount of stability is imparted to the sternum by this reefing process. The perichondria will provide for regeneration of the costal cartilages within 4 to 8 weeks. The cartilage segments, although irregular, should extend straight between the end of the rib and the edge of the sternum.

It is not necessary to reef the perichondrium of the lower "floating" ribs that do not attach to the sternum.

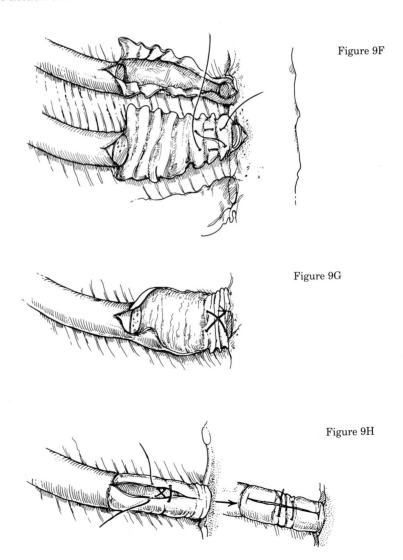

Figure 9F

Figure 9G

Figure 9H

An intercostal block is performed using 0.5% bupivacaine hydrochloride (Marcaine) in a dose of 0.3 ml/kg. This has proved quite effective for early postoperative pain control. Older patients are often placed on patient-controlled analgesia (PCA). Absorbable sutures are used for the muscle fascia, placing chest drainage tubes at the lateralmost portion of the wound to remove any blood or serum that may accumulate postoperatively (Fig. 9*I*). Subcuticular closure of the wound with Steri-Strips makes for the most cosmetic closure. Chest drains are usually left in place for 2 days, and the patient is discharged on the third or fourth postoperative day. We insist on the patient wearing a clavicular splint for 6 weeks to 3 months. Two splints are furnished to each patient so that one may be washed while the other is being worn. They are removed only for bathing.

Complications include wound infection, which may be minimized by placing the patient on antibiotics during the hospitalization period. Recurrent pectus excavatum to a degree that is likely to interfere with pulmonary expansion is seen in about 4% of patients. We have not personally reoperated on any malformations, but at least one patient benefited from substernal placement of a strut, without additional cartilage manipulation.

The objective of an operation for pectus excavatum is to enlarge the chest cavity, and therefore procedures that merely fill in the space by subcutaneous or subfascial maneuvers are only cosmetic. Pectus carinatum deformities do not produce chest volume restrictions, but they are often associated with extreme discomfort when the deformed cartilages or sternum encounter pressure. The results of pectus carinatum repair are often not as satisfactory as the results of pectus excavatum repair, because very often these deformities are asymmetric and the sternum is twisted, making perfect sternal alignment difficult. It is even more difficult to ensure that it will heal in that position. The principles of surgical repair of pectus carinatum are the same as those for pectus excavatum repair. To minimize the possibility of a recurrent deformity, pectus carinatum should be repaired after the patient has gone through the adolescent growth spurt.

References

Shamberger RC, Welch KJ: Surgical repair of pectus excavatum. J Pediatr Surg 23:615–622, 1988.
Shamberger RC, Welch KJ, Castaneda AR, et al: Anterior chest wall deformities and congenital heart disease. J Thorac Cardiovasc Surg 96:427–432, 1988.

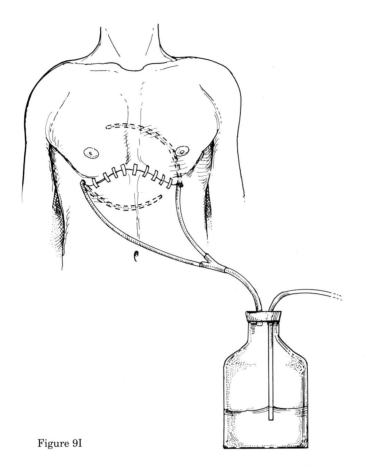

Figure 9I

CHAPTER 10

Esophageal atresia/ Tracheoesophageal fistula

The various forms of esophageal atresia/tracheoesophageal fistula (Fig. 10*A*) may be associated with prematurity or with any of a constellation of defects known as the VACTERL (*v*ertebral, *a*nal, *c*ardiac, *t*racheal, *e*sophageal, *r*enal, and *l*imb) association. The surgical approach to the esophagus and the tracheoesophageal fistula must be coordinated with the need to palliate or treat a heart defect. In the 1960s we recommended "staging" for infants weighing less than 2 kg, but currently we will do an esophageal repair on an infant who weighs as little as 1300 gm. Some ill infants with heart defects require staging by division and suture of the fistula, without esophageal anastomosis, during repair of a coarctation or a patent ductus arteriosus.

Pneumonitis—either chemical or bacterial—remains a serious preoperative consideration.

Preoperatively the patient with the most common type of esophageal atresia with distal tracheoesophageal fistula is nursed in a semiupright position with a No. 10 French sump suction catheter (Argyle catheter) in the proximal esophageal pouch (Fig. 10*B*).

General endotracheal anesthesia is used. A No. 18 to 22 French red rubber catheter should be placed into the upper esophageal pouch for easier delineation of the upper esophagus. The patient is positioned as for a right thoracotomy (Fig. 10*C*). We prefer an extrapleural approach through the fourth intercostal space or bed of the fourth rib. The chest wall incision may use the standard posterolateral thoracotomy approach with transection of the latissimus dorsi and serratus anterior muscles or the muscle sparing approach in which these two large muscles are retracted anteriorly and the fourth intercostal space reached through the triangle of auscultation. The intercostal muscles are carefully divided and the plane of the endothoracic fascia is developed. The pleural dissection is carried superiorly to the apex of the chest and inferiorly for a couple of interspaces. Posteriorly, the dissection is carried around to the vertebral bodies. The two highest intercostal veins are divided, and the azygos is reflected anteriorly with the pleura.

The vagus nerve is identified on reaching the mediastinum. Below the atretic segment, the vagus helps in identification of the distal esophageal segment.

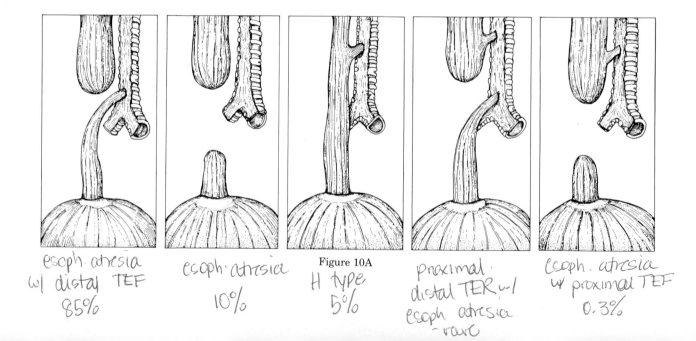

esoph. atresia w/ distal TEF 85%

esoph. atresia 10%

Figure 10A

H type 5%

proximal distal TEF w/ esoph atresia - rare

esoph. atresia w proximal TEF 0.3%

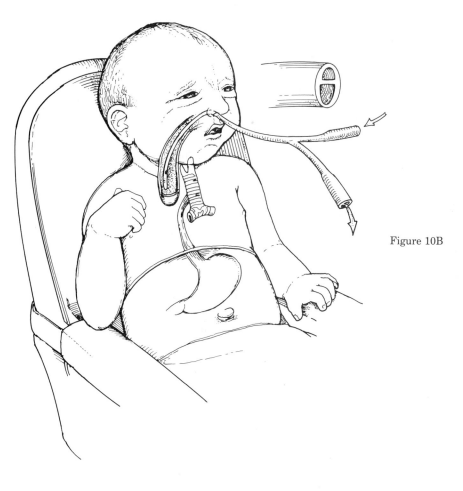

Figure 10B

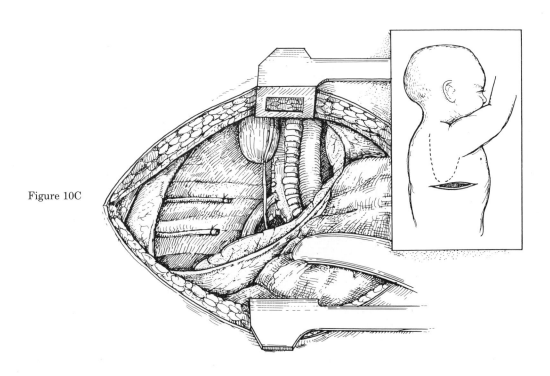

Figure 10C

The distal esophagus is identified and looped with tape and then dissected proximally to its junction with the trachea (Fig. 10*D*).

The fistula is divided just at the posterior aspect of the trachea, and the tracheal end closed with interrupted 5–0 silk sutures (Fig. 10*E*).

Identification of the upper pouch is facilitated by having the anesthesiologist push on the red rubber catheter that was passed into the proximal pouch (Fig. 10*F*). A heavy traction suture is placed into the distal end of the pouch, and the proximal pouch is dissected off the trachea as far into the neck as possible. It is important to look for a proximal pouch tracheoesophageal fistula that may not have been previously detected.

The most commonly used anastomosis uses the end-to-end, single-layer, full-thickness, interrupted suture technique (Fig. 10*G*). There is invariably a difference in the sizes of the two esophageal ends, and the sutures should be placed to account for this disparity. Fine silk, polypropylene, or monofilament absorbable suture may be used for the anastomosis. The Haight two-layer anastomosis has been employed for many years in an effort to reduce the incidence of anastomotic leaks (Fig. 10*H*). The tunica muscularis of the upper pouch is dissected free from the mucosa for a distance of about 1 cm. The full thickness of the lower segment is sutured to the mucosa of the upper segment as the first layer. The tunica muscularis of the upper pouch is then pulled down over the inner suture line, and the muscle layers are approximated to cover the inner anastomotic layer. After the anterior outer layer of sutures are positioned, the esophagus is rotated, and the posterior sutures are placed.

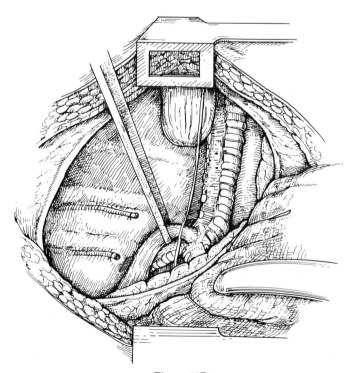

Figure 10D

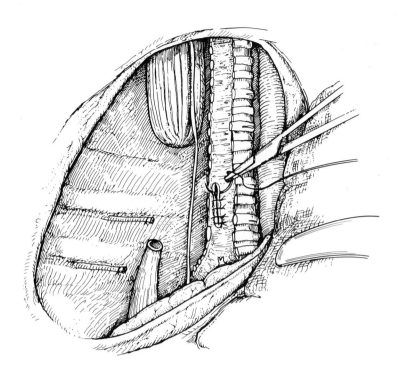

Figure 10E

Figure 10F

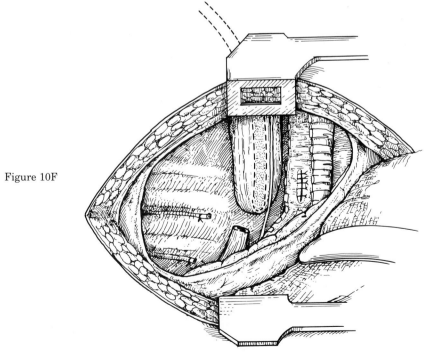

A retropleural chest tube is sutured to the intercostal or perivertebral fascia so that the tube does not touch the anastomosis. The wound is then closed in anatomic layers (Fig. 10I).

Surgical treatment of esophageal atresia that does not involve a distal tracheoesophageal fistula usually involves esophageal substitution (see Chapter 31). A gastrostomy is established in the newborn for feeding (see Chapter 13), and the definitive procedure is planned after the child is older than 1 month.

Division and suture of the isolated tracheoesophageal fistula without esophageal atresia is most commonly done through a right cervical approach. This operative procedure is facilitated by bronchoscopic placement of a ureteral catheter through the fistula. The distal end of this catheter is retrieved from the esophagus and used as a traction device by the anesthesiologist to aid in elevation and identification of the fistula. The divided ends of the fistula are closed with interrupted suture and the esophagus is rotated slightly to prevent apposition of the suture lines. Some adjacent tissue may be interposed between them. Drains are not used.

The major early postoperative complications after repair of esophageal atresia/tracheoesophageal fistula are atelectasis and pneumonitis. Respiratory therapy must be carried out cautiously, as overzealous suctioning may injure a suture line.

Anastomotic leak may complicate the postoperative period. We leave the chest tube in place for 10 days, because some leaks have occurred as late as 9 days postoperatively.

Gastroesophageal reflux is common after esophageal atresia/tracheoesophageal fistula repair and may produce anastomotic stricture or nutritional disturbance. About 35% of these patients will require fundoplication as therapy for gastroesophageal reflux.

Reference

Holder TM: Esophageal atresia and tracheoesophageal malformations. In Ashcraft KW, Holder TM, eds: Pediatric Surgery. 2nd ed. Philadelphia, WB Saunders, 1993, pp 249–269.

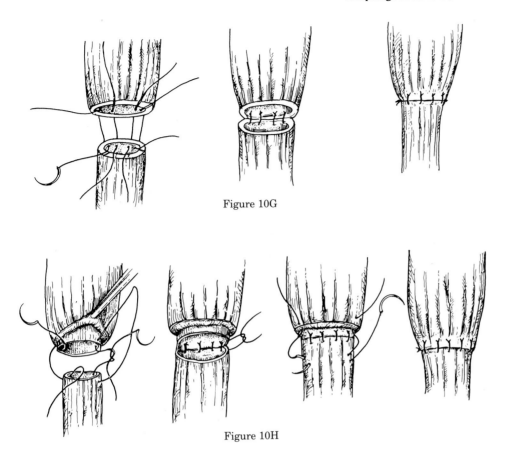

Figure 10G

Figure 10H

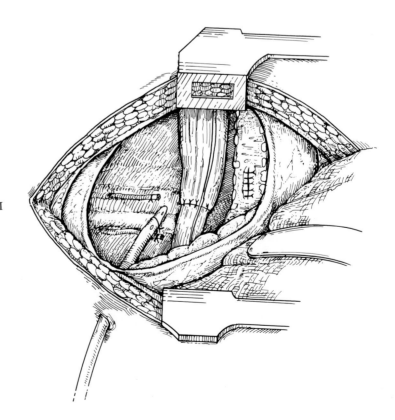

Figure 10I

CHAPTER

11

Mediastinal lesions

Probably the most common lesion occuring in the mediastinum is a neuroblastoma or ganglioneuroma in the paravertebral area. Most of these are discovered incidentally when a child has a chest radiograph for respiratory disease (Fig. 11A). They may be located anywhere from the apex of the chest down to the lower portion of the mediastinum, even extending through the diaphragm and into the abdominal cavity.

These lesions arise from the paravertebral sympathetic chain but may extend via the intercostal nerve roots through the foramina into the spinal canal. Preoperative evaluation requires careful study of the region by computed tomographic (CT) scan or magnetic resonance imaging. If the lesion does extend through the neural foramina into the spinal canal, laminectomy along with removal of the intraspinal portion is advisable before surgical attack on the mediastinal lesion because of the potential for postoperative edema resulting in spinal cord damage.

The lesion should be removed as completely as possible using the standard posterior lateral thoracotomy approach.

Lesions in the wall of the esophagus (Fig. 11B) that are in the upper portion of the mediastinum are most often esophageal duplication cysts. Lesions in the lower part of the mediastinum are most often bronchogenic cysts. Both types of lesions share a common muscular wall with the lumen of the esophagus (Fig. 11B, inset), which means that the best way to remove them is to open the muscular coat and strip out the mucosa of the cyst without trying to resect all of the muscle coats.

Hilar adenopathy is often associated with histoplasmosis but may result from bacterial infection as well (Fig. 11C). These lesions are often discovered on radiographs and can be further delineated by CT. When they occur in children, there is some concern that they may be evidence of a lymphoma. A definitive diagnosis is best established by nodal excision or biopsy; this may be done by open thoracotomy or thoracoscopy with biopsy.

The most acutely life-threatening of all the mediastinal lesions is the anteriorly located thymic lesion, which can produce severe airway compression (Fig. 11D). These are usually lymphomas, which can enlarge very rapidly, and patients are usually in their teens. Shortness of breath, especially when lying supine, is the major symptom. A precise stem cell tissue diagnosis for definitive chemotherapy is usually not possible, as these patients must maintain a sitting position to be able to breathe. General anesthesia is very dangerous. The safest course of action in these patients is pretreatment with corticosteroids, which produce very rapid shrinkage of the tumor. Unfortunately, however, steroid therapy often makes precise histologic determination of the type of malignancy difficult, if not impossible. In most cases, after pretreatment with steroids, surgical biopsy or thymectomy is not done. The tumors are so responsive to both steroids and chemotherapy that surgical removal adds nothing to the outcome.

The thymus is sometimes removed for treatment of myasthenia gravis. The response to thymectomy is best in girls whose symptoms are of recent onset and who have responded well to medical therapy. Total thymectomy may be accomplished through either a right or left fourth interspace thoracotomy or a sternal splitting approach. Thoracoscopic thymectomy has also been reported.

Teratomas may occur in the anterior mediastinum. These tumors are far more slow growing than thymic malignancies and do not pose the anesthetic risk of thymic tumors. Therefore, standard thoracotomy is advised for removal of these lesions. They are usually benign and do not require resection of any important mediastinal structures.

Reference

Pokorny WJ: Mediastinal tumors. In Ashcraft KW, Holder TM, eds: Pediatric Surgery. 2nd ed. Philadelphia, WB Saunders, 1993, pp 218–227.

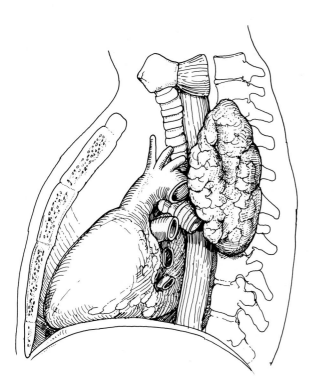

Figure 11A

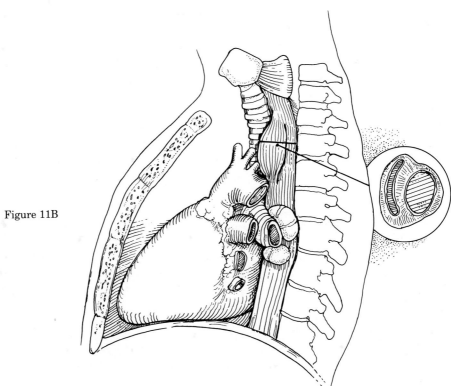

Figure 11B

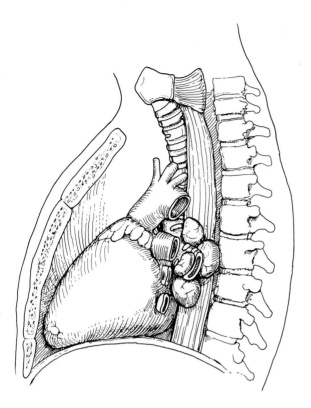

Figure 11C

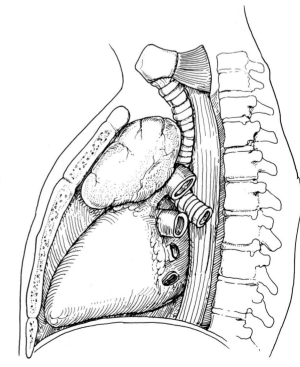

Figure 11D

Colon interposition

Esophageal substitution by colon interposition is usually done in pediatric patients who have esophageal atresia or a caustic stricture. Most patients will have a gastrostomy in place (Fig. 12A); patients with esophageal atresia usually have a cervical esophagostomy as well. The two most common approaches are to use the left colon through the left chest or the right colon in a substernal interposition.

For the left colon interposition, the patient is positioned for a left thoracotomy. The chest, abdomen, and neck are prepped, and a posterolateral sixth or seventh intercostal space incision is made (Fig. 12B). The diaphragm is opened and the abdomen entered through either a curved incision placed laterally and close to the ribs or by a radial incision (Fig. 12C). Alternatively, a separate abdominal incision may be used for the abdominal portion of the procedure. The transverse and left colon are freed, and the blood supply is assessed. The left marginal branch of the middle colic artery is temporarily occluded to determine whether the colonic segment will remain viable based on the left colic artery. If the blood supply is adequate, the colon and the marginal vessels are divided at the level of the previous occlusion (Fig. 12D).

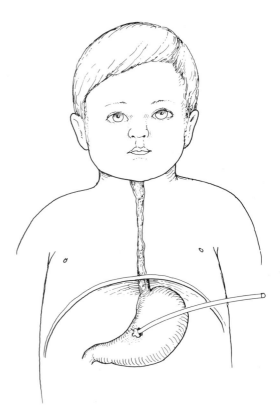

Figure 12*A*

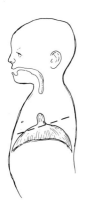

Figure 12*B*

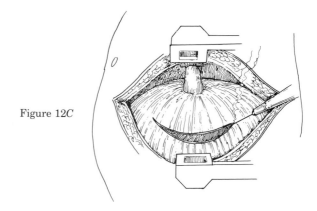

Figure 12*C*

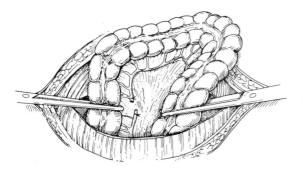

Figure 12*D*

Distally the colon is divided a suitable distance to provide adequate length to bridge the esophageal gap. The continuity of the colon is re-established by an end-to-end anastomosis of the transverse colon to the descending colon. The spleen and pancreas are reflected anteriorly so that the colon segment and its blood supply will pass behind them. An incision is made near the hiatus, through which the colon segment and its blood supply are passed into the chest (Fig. 12*E*). The colon is sutured to the distal esophagus using two layers of interrupted sutures (Fig. 12*F*). The inner layer consists of mucosa sutured to mucosa, and the outer layer consists of esophageal musculature sutured to the seromuscular layer of the colon. The proximal end of the colon conduit is trimmed to length so that there is no redundancy. The proximal anastomosis may be constructed in the neck or in the chest; it is similar to the distal anastomosis (Fig. 12*G*).

Figures 12*A* through 12*I* and 12*K* through 12*M* are from Ashcraft KW, Holder TM, eds. Pediatric Surgery. 2nd ed. Philadelphia, WB Saunders, 1993.

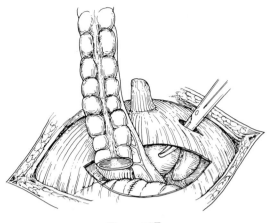

Figure 12E

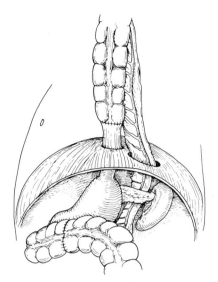

Figure 12F

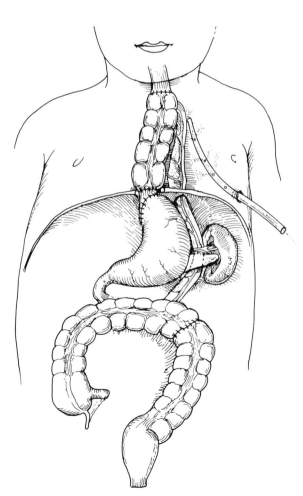

Figure 12G

In some instances there is not sufficient distal esophagus for an anastomosis. In these cases the colon may be brought down through the hiatus and the anastomosis made to the posterior aspect of the body of the stomach (Figs. 12*H*, 12*I*).

For the substernal colon interposition the patient is placed in a supine position. The neck, abdomen, and chest are included in the operative field. A vertical midline abdominal incision is made (Fig. 12*J*) and the right colon mobilized. The vessels of the right colon are temporarily occluded, basing the blood supply of the right and transverse colon on the middle colic artery. If the blood supply is satisfactory, the ileum is divided just proximal to the ileocecal valve, and the transverse colon is divided just to the left of the middle colic artery (Fig. 12*K*). The continuity of the colon is established by end-to-end anastomosis of the terminal ileum to the transverse colon. The colon and its pedicle are then passed in isoperistolic fashion behind the stomach and through the lesser omentum (Fig. 12*L*). A substernal tunnel is created by blunt dissection, staying close to the sternum and reflecting the pleura to either side. It is important that the tunnel be wide enough that the colon can be passed without much traction being necessary. The proximal end of the colon is temporarily closed, and the suture is left long so that it can be used to pull the segment through the tunnel. The colon is then trimmed both proximally and distally so that it bridges the gap between the proximal esophagus and the stomach without redundancy or kinking. The proximal end is anastomosed to the esophagus, and the distal end is sutured to the body of the stomach (Fig. 12*M*). Attempts to make a valve mechanism to prevent reflux have been without uniform success. A pyloroplasty promotes gastric emptying and may reduce reflux.

If there is any question about the blood supply to the proximal colon, the anastomosis is delayed. Usually it is possible to proceed with end-to-end anastomosis between the proximal esophagus and the proximal colon. A two-layered interrupted anastomosis is preferred.

References

Waterston DJ: Replacement of oesophagus with colon in childhood. In Rob C, Smith R, eds: Operative Surgery. Vol 2. 2nd ed. London, Butterworths, 1968, pp 367–374.
Azar H, Chrispin AR, Waterston DJ: Esophageal replacement with transverse colon infants and children. J Pediatr Surg 6:3–9, 1971.

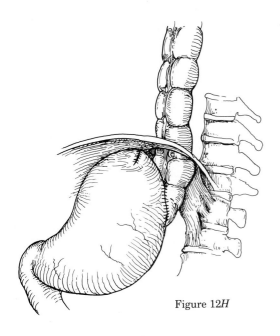

Figure 12*H*

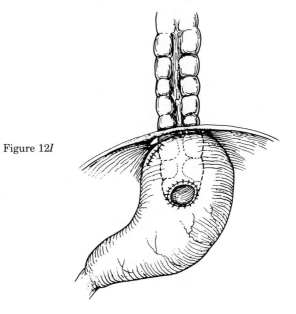

Figure 12*I*

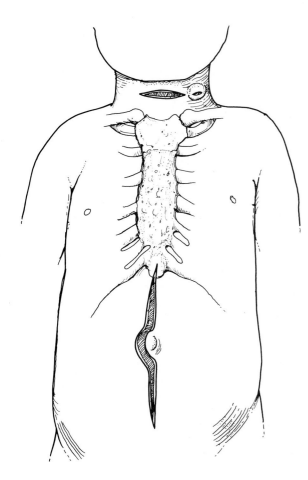

Figure 12*J*

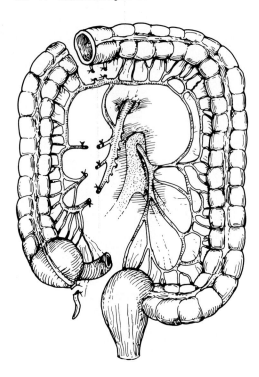

Figure 12K

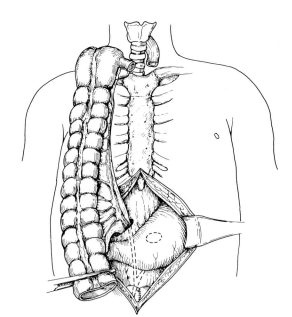

Figure 12L

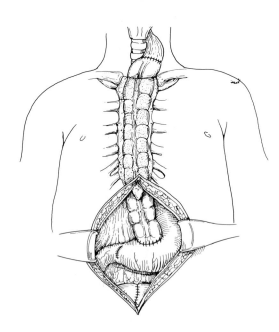

Figure 12M

13

Reversed gastric tube

A reversed gastric tube may be used to replace part or all of the esophagus. It is usually performed through a left thoracoabdominal incision or through separate abdominal and left thoracic incisions. Through the upper abdominal incision, the stomach and its blood supply are assessed. The reversed gastric tube receives its main blood supply from the gastroepiploic vessels, and these must remain intact. If trial occlusion of the right gastroepiploic artery reveals good pulses, the artery is divided as far distally as practical. The omentum is divided, preserving the gastroepiploic vessel on which the greater curvature gastric tube will be hinged (Fig. 13A).

An incision is then made in the greater curvature at the point of division of the gastroepiploic artery and at right angles to the greater curvature of the stomach, extending as far onto the stomach as is necessary to provide a tube of adequate size. The antral side of this incision is then closed either by suture or staples. The tube is then created along the greater curvature using a GIA stapler (Fig. 13B). The use of a large Robinson catheter along the greater curvature forms a mandrel guiding the placement of the GIA stapler to ensure a uniform tube and an adequate lumen; a No. 36 French tube is about the right size for a toddler. The short gastric vessels are preserved.

The gastric tube is developed up to about the level of the fundus or as far as is required to bridge the esophageal gap. The cut surface of the staple line may be reinforced with suture, but this probably is not necessary. The esophagus to be replaced is then freed through the hiatus as far as possible. The gastroesophageal junction is transected and closed by either staples or suture. The remainder of the "bad" esophagus is removed. The tube is then folded proximally across the body of the stomach and threaded through the hiatus. The plication of the fundus to the gastric tube prevents reflux. The tube is then anastomosed to the esophagus using interrupted sutures (Fig. 13C). If the anastomosis is to be done at the level of the aortic arch, it may be necessary to deliver the esophagus from the mediastinum and create the anasto-

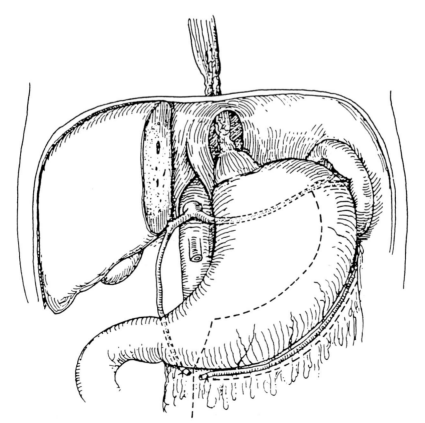

Figure 13A

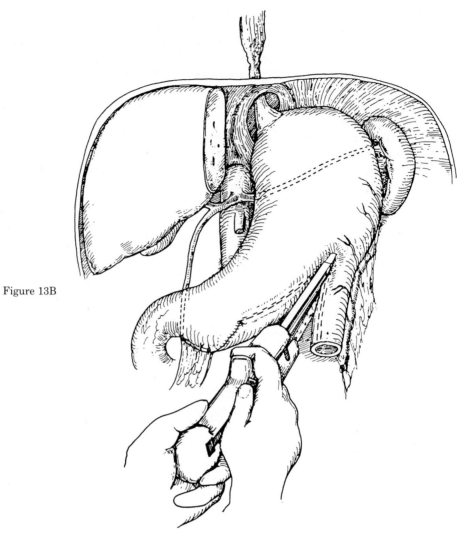

Figure 13B

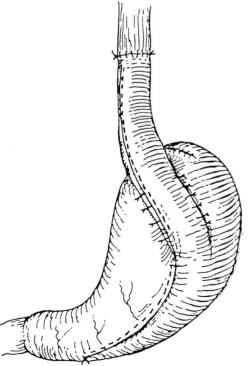

Figure 13C

mosis to the left of the arch. The stomach should be decompressed by gastrostomy or by a nasogastric tube placed at the time of operation. The tube is removed as soon as gastric emptying is demonstrated.

Most patients requiring a reversed gastric tube for esophageal substitution will already have undergone a gastrostomy. Placement of the gastrostomy on the greater curve of the stomach may preclude the use of a gastric tube. It is always best to place a gastrostomy performed for any reason nearer to the lesser curve than the greater curve.

The major complication of gastric tube interposition is reflux, which will produce anastomotic stricture or esophageal ulcers. Placement of the tube through the esophageal hiatus and the posterior fundoplication will minimize reflux.

References

Anderson KD, Randolph JG: The gastric tube for esophageal replacement in children. J Thorac Cardiovasc Surg 66:333–342, 1973.

Ashcraft KW: The esophagus. In Ashcraft KW, Holder TM, eds: Pediatric Surgery. 2nd ed. Philadelphia, WB Saunders, 1993, pp 228–248.

All figures in this chapter are from Ashcraft KW: Esophageal atresia and tracheoesophageal fistula. Chest Surg Clin North Am 3(3):477–493, 1993.

CHAPTER

14

Congenital diaphragmatic hernia

For many neonates with diaphragmatic hernia, correction of the defect is the easiest part of their care. The most challenging aspect is postoperative cardiopulmonary support. However, the repair involves some important considerations.

The operative approach should be through the abdomen. For a left-sided hernia a left upper quadrant transverse incision is made just below the rib cage (Fig. 14A). With a small retractor under the anterior edge of the diaphragmatic defect, gentle traction on the abdominal viscera will usually allow the viscera to be withdrawn from the chest onto the anterior abdominal wall. The stomach, the spleen, part of the pancreas, the small bowel, and the proximal colon are often in the chest (Fig. 14B). The posterior aspect of the defect is covered by peritoneum. An incision is made in the peritoneum posteriorly and the posterior muscular edge freed to develop as much posterior diaphragm as possible (Fig. 14C). Much of the time it is possible to carry out direct closure. The one found to be most secure is a vest-over-pants closure using horizontal mattress sutures as the first row and then a simple suture between each of these to reinforce the first suture line (Fig. 14D, inset). In patients in whom the defect is so large that direct approximation cannot be accomplished, the diaphragm is patched with a sheet of Dacron, Gore-Tex, or

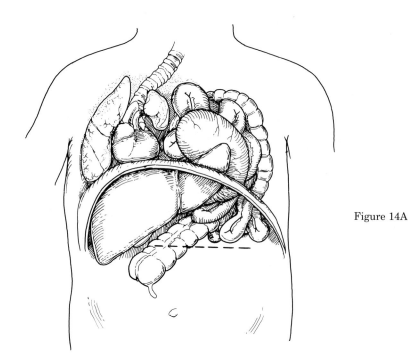

Figure 14A

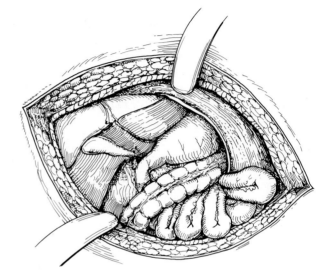

Figure 14B

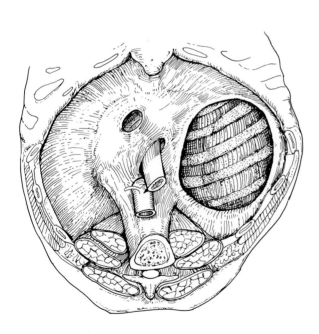

Figure 14C

mesh using continuous nonabsorbable sutures (Fig. 14*D*). The lateral rim may be absent, making it necessary to put the lateral sutures either around the rib or into the intercostal muscle.

A chest tube is left in place for water-seal drainage only. Active suction may pull the mediastinum so far to the ipsilateral side that the better lung is made emphysematous (Fig. 14*E*). An umbilical artery catheter is very helpful in ventilator or extracorporeal membrane oxygenation (ECMO) management. A gastrostomy usually provides the most effective gastric decompression. Although these critically ill infants have a malrotation, we do not routinely perform Ladd's procedure. The viscera are returned to the abdominal cavity. Wound closure may be difficult, because the peritoneal cavity is small; on occasion, a Silastic gusset is required for abdominal wound closure. Primary closure in layers is usually possible.

Complications most often relate to pulmonary hypoplasia, persistent pulmonary hypertension, or both. Much controversy exists with regard to the best preoperative and postoperative management.

Reference

de Lorimier AA: Diaphragmatic hernia. In Ashcraft KW, Holder TM, eds: Pediatric Surgery. 2nd ed. Philadelphia, WB Saunders, 1993, pp 204–217.

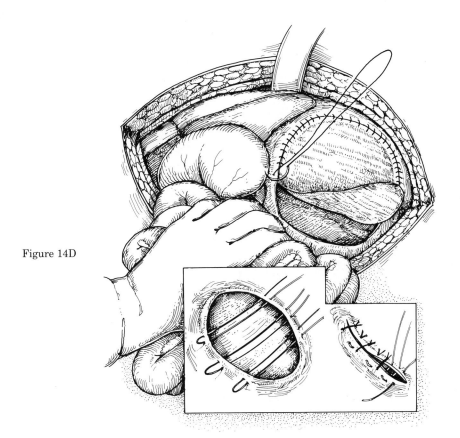

Figure 14D

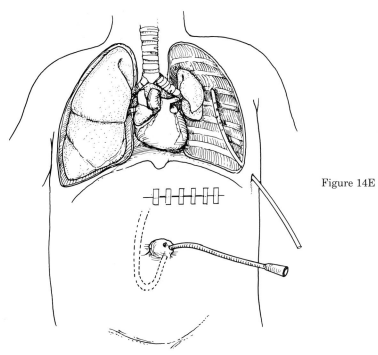

Figure 14E

CHAPTER

15

Fundoplication

The near epidemic of gastroesophageal (GE) reflux in children since the 1970s has been largely a result of the widespread recognition of the protean manifestations that GE reflux can produce in children. These include recurrent pneumonitis, croup, cough, choking, and well-documented instances of acute life-threatening events or sudden infant death syndrome. The reflux of acid into the lower esophagus can produce esophagitis with severe heartburn; ulceration, with replacement of esophageal mucosa by gastric mucosa (Barrett's esophagus); or distal esophageal stricture. The nutritional manifestations of GE reflux are seen most commonly in patients with mental or motor retardation, but they also occur in normal children. The loss of caloric intake because of reflux is so significant that failure to thrive or even marasmus may develop in some infants. The relationship between GE reflux and neurologic impairment is as yet incompletely explained. In some institutions that treat pediatric patients, the vast majority of patients requiring fundoplication for GE reflux are those with neurologic impairment.

The diagnosis of GE reflux is made only after the pediatrician or surgeon realizes that reflux may be the cause of the patient's disorder. A barium study to delineate the anatomy is extremely important. This may show an esophageal stricture, a hiatal hernia with gastric rugae above the level of the diaphragm, or gastric outlet obstruction such as malrotation with Ladd's bands. An experienced radiologist can usually discern pathologic GE reflux from the physiologic reflux seen on the upper gastrointestinal (GI) study. A 30-minute delayed abdominal film that shows barium in the stomach and well down into the small bowel is very helpful. If barium is seen in the esophagus on this study, GE reflux is usually present. The most definitive diagnostic test for GE reflux is the 24-hour pH study. The derived score will separate normal amounts of postprandial reflux from the pathologic reflux that occurs later. The percentage of time in which the pH is below 4 is important, because this is the process that produces esophagitis. It must be remembered that a patient whose acid production is being inhibited by medication or who is taking heavy doses of antacid may not have enough acid to register on a 24-hour pH study, even though massive GE reflux is present.

There is no known medical treatment that will cure the anatomic disorder that produces GE reflux. Medications that alter esophageal and gastric motility and gastric acid production and promote gastric emptying may ameliorate the symptoms and allow the patient to live with reflux, but, particularly in children, a lifetime program of medications is sometimes dangerous and is often not followed.

Surgical treatment of GE reflux is perhaps more effective in children than in adults, and therefore, operative treatment seems to be used more often for pediatric patients with significant GE reflux. All fundoplication operative procedures depend on the establishment of an intra-abdominal portion of esophagus coupled with plication of the stomach to the lower esophagus so that an angle of His is established. These two comprise the valve mechanism. The most commonly performed operative procedure is the 360-degree wrap described by Nissen. We prefer the 180-degree wrap described by Thal. It has the same success rate as the Nissen procedure, allows 99% of patients to burp or vomit, and carries fewer complications in terms of serious "gas bloats" and intestinal obstruction.

All figures in this chapter are from Ashcraft KW: Gastroesophageal reflux. In Ashcraft KW, Holder TM, eds: Pediatric Surgery. 2nd ed. Philadelphia, WB Saunders, 1993, pp 278–280.

THAL FUNDOPLICATION

We prefer a transverse upper abdominal incision, because the transverse colon helps to prevent small bowel protrusion through the wound. This factor probably is responsible for the low incidence of adhesive small bowel obstruction in our series. The brevity of the procedure when compared with the Nissen fundoplication also may play a part in reducing postoperative intestinal complications. The upper edge of the wound is retracted cephalad, the liver grasped with the surgeon's left hand, and the membranous attachment of the left lobe of the liver taken down from the underside of the diaphragm (Fig. 15A). Care must be taken to prevent injury to the hepatic veins. The liver is then turned downward, protected by a sponge, and retracted to the patient's right.

The peritoneum overlying the esophagus at the GE junction is then incised transversely (Fig. 15B), and blunt dissection is used to expose the lower portion of the esophagus.

We prefer to pass a blunt dissector behind the esophagus from the patient's right to the patient's left, grasping a Dacron tape at that point and pulling it through for traction purposes (Fig. 15C). Care is taken to include both the anterior and the posterior vagus nerves with the esophagus during this maneuver. An appropriate length of esophagus is mobilized anteriorly, laterally, and posteriorly so that this portion of the esophagus can be established into the abdominal cavity as part of the valve mechanism (Fig. 15D).

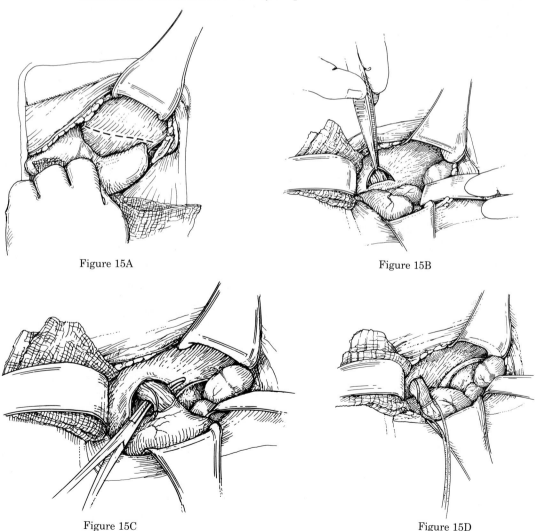

Figure 15A

Figure 15B

Figure 15C

Figure 15D

The exposed esophagus is lifted by a small retractor and retracted to the left so that the hiatus is exposed. The overlarge hiatus is closed with a figure-of-8 2-0 or 3-0 silk suture, ensuring that good "bites" are obtained of the crura and that the ligature is not tied so tightly that necrosis will result in a recurrent hiatal hernia (Fig. 15E). This "limiting stitch" is then attached to the posterior wall of the esophagus, being careful to avoid entrapment of the posterior vagus nerve. This fixes the lower esophagus within the abdominal cavity and aids in the prevention of GE reflux (Fig. 15F).

The limbs of the Dacron tape, which have been held in one clamp, are then separated so that the anterior portion of the stomach may be mobilized to apply to the anterior half of the esophagus (Fig. 15G). The surface area of the stomach exceeds that of this portion of the esophagus, making for a "floppy" fundoplication. The fundoplication is carried out by using a continuous suture, beginning at the greater curve GE junction and extending up the left side of the esophagus, bringing the fundus upward (Fig. 15H). As the level of the hiatus is reached, the suture includes the stomach, esophagus, and hiatus (Fig. 15I). The suture line is then turned toward the patient's right. After reaching the right lateral portion of the esophagus, the suture line turns to go down to the GE junction on the lesser curved side where this suture is tied (Fig. 15J).

At this point, the anterior wall of the intra-abdominal esophagus is covered by upper stomach (Fig. 15K). We use a nasogastric tube to provide stability for the esophagus during the creation of this fundoplication, but its size in no way determines the tightness or looseness of the fundoplication. The Dacron tape and the nasogastric tube are removed at this time, and the wound is closed. Feedings of liquids begin the following morning, progressing very rapidly to a diet appropriate for age. The usual hospital stay is 48 hours.

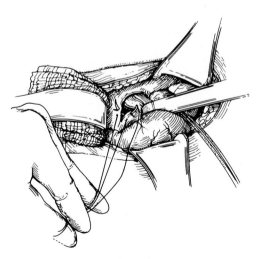

Figure 15E

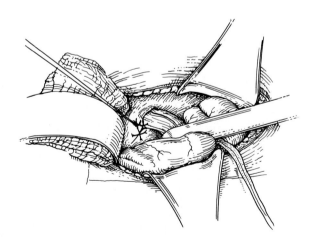

Figure 15F

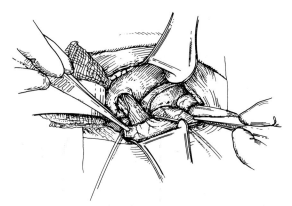

Figure 15G

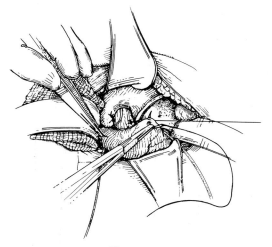

Figure 15H

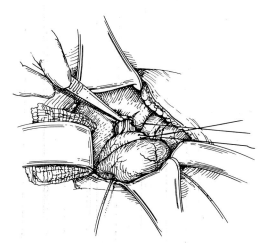

Figure 15I

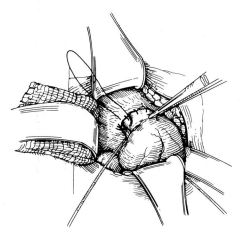

Figure 15J

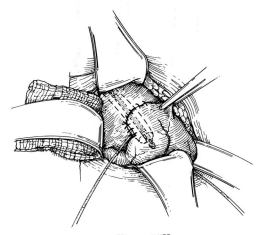

Figure 15K

NISSEN FUNDOPLICATION

The Nissen fundoplication initially is carried out in the same manner as the Thal fundoplication just described in that the esophagus is dissected free of the hiatus and the hiatus is closed posteriorly with permanent suture. We usually divide the upper short gastric vessels to allow adequate mobilization of the stomach. A sizable bougie is placed in the patient's esophagus for the procedure to ensure that the wrap is not made so tightly that obstruction to the passage of food occurs (Fig. 15L). The fundus is then drawn around behind the esophagus (Fig. 15M), and interrupted sutures are used to construct the 360-degree wrap (Fig. 15N). These sutures include the seromuscular portion of the stomach on the left, a bite of esophagus well away from the anterior vagus nerve, and a seromuscular stitch in the stomach on the right. When these sutures are tied, a cuff is formed around the lower esophagus, much like a blood pressure cuff (Fig. 15O). Distention of the stomach creates a valve that acts very much like a blood pressure cuff and can completely shut off the lower esophagus (Fig. 15P).

The fact that the Nissen fundoplication will preclude eructation and vomiting in the vast majority of patients leads to one of the difficulties in this procedure. In patients who swallow air, acute gastric distention (known as the "gas bloat" syndrome) can occur; gastric necrosis, rupture, and death have been known to result. Some surgeons add a venting gastrostomy to all patients under the age of 3 years to allow decompression of the stomach.

COMPLICATIONS

Complications may occur with both types of fundoplication. Postoperative edema may result in distal esophageal swelling and the inability to ingest solid foods for a period of time. This edema may be troublesome for up to 4 weeks in patients who have had esophagitis.

The gas bloat syndrome, which has occurred in only 2 of 1300 patients undergoing the Thal fundoplication in our series, is much more common in patients who have had Nissen fundoplication and may result in the need for temporary nasogastric decompression.

The incidence of postoperative small bowel adhesive obstruction appears to be less with the Thal procedure than with the Nissen procedure, primarily because of the shorter operative time and less exposure needed for the Thal fundoplication.

A slipped Nissen fundoplication will produce a bilobed stomach, which sometimes is more obstructive than the intact Nissen fundoplication. Breakdown of the Thal fundoplication has been seen in approximately 1.8% of the patients in our series. Recurrent hiatal hernia, which initially was seen in about the same percentage of patients, has diminished in incidence, because we now place the "limiting stitch" even in those patients whose hiatus is not deemed to be overlarge.

Long-term follow-up of the Thal fundoplication in our series is currently at a maximum of about 18 years, with almost all recurrences being seen within the first year. Fundoplications done in infants are known to have grown with the patient, and very satisfactory control of reflux has been accomplished.

Reference

Ashcraft KW: Gastroesophageal reflux. In Ashcraft KW, Holder TM, eds: Pediatric Surgery. 2nd ed. Philadelphia, WB Saunders, 1993, pp 270–288.

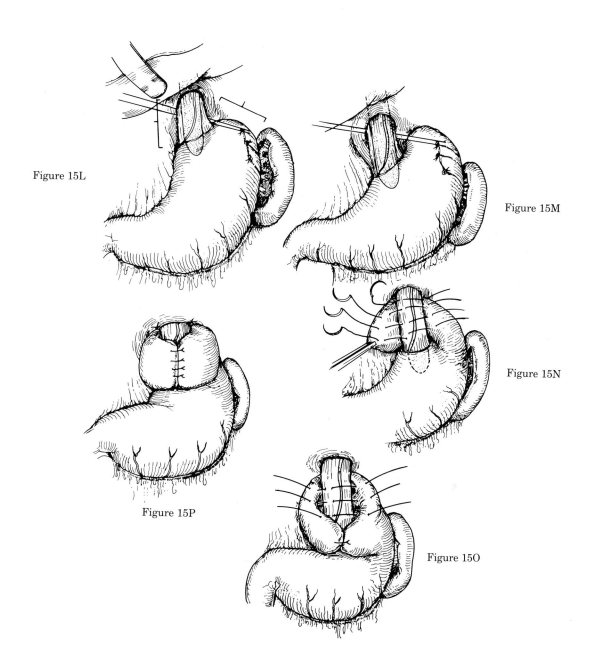

Figure 15L

Figure 15M

Figure 15N

Figure 15P

Figure 15O

CHAPTER

16

Achalasia

Achalasia is a disease of unknown etiology in which the distal esophagus becomes obstructed by hypertrophied muscle. If it goes unrecognized and untreated, megaesophagus with tortuosity can occur. The patient will ingest food and regurgitate it, sometimes hours later, without evidence of its having reached the stomach. Malnutrition is common.

The diagnosis is made by barium study. The barium column will come to a point before entry into the stomach, and there may be vastly delayed emptying of the esophagus into the stomach. Esophageal motility by manometric studies has shown diminution in prograde peristalsis, with only tertiary contractions in patients with long-standing achalasia.

There is no medical treatment for achalasia. Bougienage sometimes results in temporary relief of symptoms but often does not. Children who have achalasia usually do not have an esophagus that is exceedingly dilated or whose motility is severely disturbed. Early surgical treatment of achalasia in children is urged.

HELLER MYOTOMY/THAL FUNDOPLICATION

Our preference for the surgical treatment of achalasia is to perform a Heller myotomy anteriorly, accompanied by an anterior fundoplication as described in Chapter 15. A transverse abdominal incision is used, and the lower esophagus is exposed (Fig. 16A). Care is taken to protect the vagus nerves throughout the myotomy and the fundoplication.

The distal esophagus will be found to be thick and rigid. An instrument is passed from the patient's right to the patient's left behind the esophagus (Fig. 16B). A Dacron tape is then passed behind the esophagus to be used for traction, while the lower esophagus is mobilized bluntly from the hiatus and the lower mediastinum (Fig. 16C). The outer longitudinal muscle and inner circular muscle are then incised anteriorly, care being taken not to enter the lumen of the esophagus. The submucosa is dissected from the inside of this thickened esophageal muscle so that the myotomy gapes in much the same way as a myotomy for pyloric stenosis. The myotomy is carried cephalad only as far as the fundoplication is to be constructed and is carried distally onto the stomach, past the serosal reflection, so that the upper gastric sling does not contribute to continued obstruction (Fig. 16D and inset).

The esophagus is then lifted and the hiatus narrowed posteriorly with a figure-of-8 suture (Fig. 16E). A fundoplication after the method of Thal is then carried out (see Figs. 15A through 15I). The completed procedure is illustrated in Figure 16F.

Postoperative complications after a Heller myotomy include continued obstruction. This may be a result of ineffective esophageal peristalsis in the patient with long-standing achalasia or of an incomplete myotomy, particularly if the upper gastric muscle fibers were not divided. Because extending the myotomy onto the gastric wall may promote gastroesophageal reflux, we combine all Heller myotomies with an anterior fundoplication. Many surgeons have objected to combining fundoplication with a myotomy in this disease entity because resistance to the passage of esophageal content into the stomach is often hampered by elevated intragastric pressure and the tightness of the wrap. These objections are not a problem with the anterior fundoplication.

Long-term follow-up of 20 patients who underwent Heller myotomy and Thal fundoplication has shown excellent results without the need for reoperation, balloon dilatation, or bougienage in any of the patients.

Reference

Vane DW, Cosby K, West K, et al: Late results following esophagomyotomy in children with achalasia. J Pediatr Surg 23:515–519, 1988.

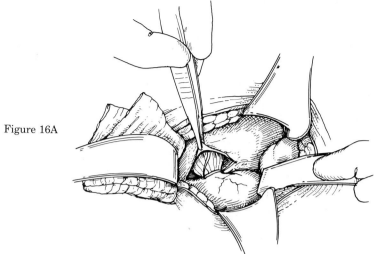

Figure 16A

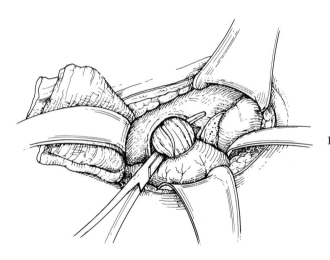

Figure 16B

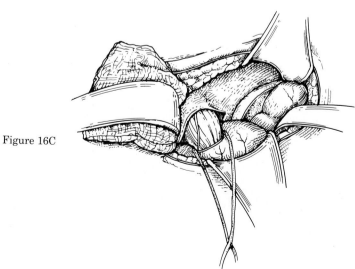

Figure 16C

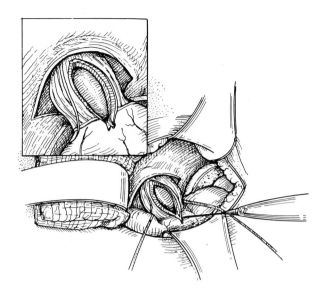

Figure 16D

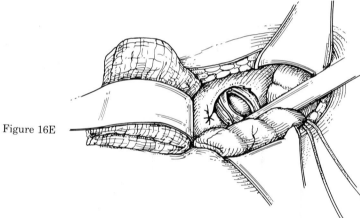

Figure 16E

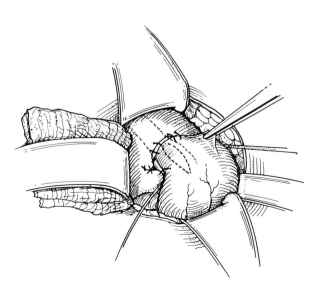

Figure 16F

17

Stamm gastrostomy

Gastrostomy is performed as an isolated procedure through either a vertical or a transverse incision made over the mid portion of the left rectus muscle 2 or 3 cm below the costal margin (a little lower in larger children) (Fig. 17A). If the tube is to be brought out through the incision, the incision need only be 1.5 to 2 cm long. If the tube is to be brought out through a separate stab incision, a larger incision will be required.

The stomach is positively identified by the short gastric vessels and the omental attachment. A site is selected on the mid portion of the body of the stomach for the gastrostomy. If a future reverse gastric tube is a possibility, the gastrostomy should be placed closer to the lessor curvature of the stomach (Fig. 17B).

The surface of the stomach is grasped with a hemostat. Two concentric pursestring sutures of silk are placed around the hemostat, the inner one being very close to the clamp and the second being out 1 cm or more to allow inversion of the stomach around the gastrostomy tube. The stomach is then opened inside the inner pursestring suture through the hemostat "track" (Fig. 17C). It may be helpful to grasp the serosa and cut through the gastric muscle with an electrocautery. The submucosa may then be grasped and the electrocautery used to enter the stomach. The electrocautery is also used to control bleeding points. The opening is then dilated with a hemostat and the gastrostomy catheter introduced. A No. 14 French catheter is satisfactory for a newborn; we prefer a de Pezzer catheter because it has a large lumen for the external diameter. It is also the most difficult catheter to dislodge, because it has no balloon to break. The shoulder helps to approximate the anterior gastric wall to the abdominal wall. The inner pursestring suture is then tied down snugly about the de Pezzer catheter. The second pursestring suture is then tied, inverting the stomach around the tube and creating a serosal tract (Fig. 17D).

If the tube is to be brought out through the incision, the stomach is incorporated in the closure of the peritoneum and posterior sheath with the pursestring sutures. If the tube is to be brought out through a stab incision, the pursestring sutures are used to attach the stomach securely to the serosa of the abdominal wall adjacent to the stab incision (Fig. 17D, inset).

The most serious complication of a gastrostomy is leak around the tube into the peritoneal cavity. This can be best prevented by "snugging" the shoulder of the tube up against the inside of the stomach and, thus, the stomach against the anterior abdominal wall. A skin suture is placed and tied around the gastrostomy tube, not to prevent the tube from falling out but to prevent it from slipping into the stomach (Fig. 17E). Slippage of the tube is also prevented by proper traction on the tube as it is taped in place (Fig. 17F).

Feeding through the gastrostomy may be started when the patient is fully recovered from the anesthesia. It is best to leave the gastrostomy suspended and open as a vent for several days to prevent gastric overdistention, which might produce a leak.

Leakage of gastric content around the tube and onto the abdominal skin is best prevented by taping the tube at a right angle to the abdominal wall. Motion of the tube promotes enlargement of the stoma. Keeping the shoulder of the de Pezzer knob against the inside of the stomach also provides a deterrent to leakage.

Granulation tissue often develops at the tube–skin interface. Silver nitrate cauterization is usually effective. Some erythema is often seen at the stoma, but infection almost never occurs.

The gastrostomy may be disrupted from the anterior abdominal wall by injudicious replacement of the tube. We allow 4 months to elapse before changing the tube for a gastrostomy button or replacing the de Pezzer cathe-

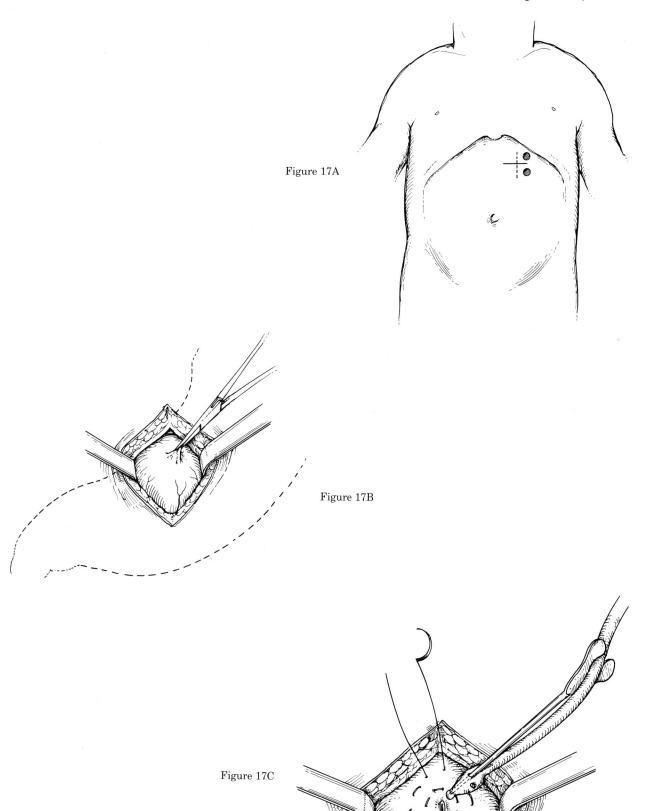

Figure 17A

Figure 17B

Figure 17C

ter. Should the gastrostomy tube become displaced during the first 2 weeks after gastrostomy creation, extreme care should be taken with replacement. This should be done either as a formal operative procedure (the safest way) or with a Foley catheter one size smaller than the original tube using fluoroscopic control, followed by instillation of contrast material to determine the tube's location and exclude an intraperitoneal leak. If a leak exists, operative placement is mandatory.

The Stamm gastrostomy is designed to close spontaneously on removal of the tube. Dislodgement of the de Pezzer catheter or of the less secure Foley balloon catheter may result in complete closure of the stoma in 6 to 8 hours. Caution is advised when replacing a gastrostomy tube.

A gastrostomy that has been in place for 6 months or longer may be complicated by the gastric mucosa lining the tract. Persistent drainage after tube removal will necessitate surgical closure.

References

Mollitt DL, Golladay ES, Seibert JJ: Symptomatic gastroesophageal reflux following gastrostomy in neurologically impaired patients. Pediatrics 75:1124–1126, 1985.

Papaila JG, Vane DW, Colville C, et al: The effect of various types of gastrostomy on the lower esophageal sphincter. J Pediatr Surg 22:1198–1202, 1987.

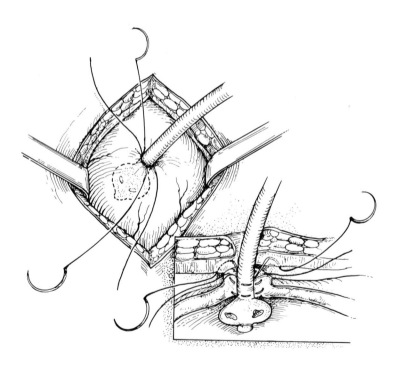

Figure 17D

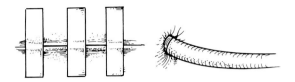

Figure 17E

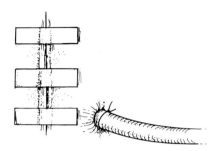

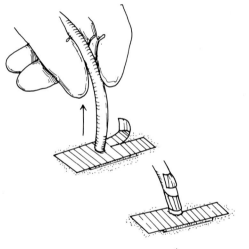

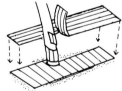

Figure 17F
Redrawn from Holder TM, Leape LL, Ashcraft KW: Gastrostomy: its use and dangers in pediatric patients. N Engl J Med 286:1345–1347, 1972. Reprinted with permission from The New England Journal of Medicine.

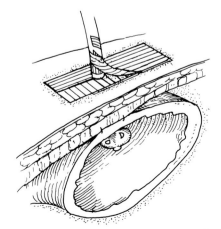

CHAPTER

18

Pyloromyotomy

Pyloromyotomy is undertaken after adequate hydration and correction of metabolic alkalosis. Before induction of anesthesia, the stomach is decompressed. No matter how long the patient may have been without oral intake, the stomach is likely to be distended with air, gastric secretions, residual feedings, or barium.

We prefer a transverse incision midway between the xiphoid and the umbilicus that extends through the skin, subcutaneous fat, and subcutaneous fascia, down to the rectus fascia and linea alba (Fig. 18A). Subcutaneous flaps are elevated deep to the subcutaneous fascia, and the peritoneal cavity is entered through a vertical linea alba incision. The antrum is grasped and retracted to the left, delivering the pylorus into the wound.

The configuration of hypertrophic pyloric stenosis is depicted in Figure 18B. The duodenal end of the pyloric sphincter ends abruptly, and the mucosa is close to the serosa at this point. The arrow indicates the most likely site of inadvertent entry into the duodenal lumen. The antral end of the pylorus is less distinct. Blood vessels originate on the superior and inferior aspects of the pylorus, which creates a relatively avascular area on the anterior surface. At the distal end of the hypertrophied musculature is the vein of Mayo and a white line that demarcates the distal end of the hypertrophied musculature. The surgeon's finger helps to delineate the distal end of the pyloric muscle (Fig. 18C). The incision is made in the more avascular area, extending through the proximal portion of the white line distally and up onto the antrum proximally. It is safer to begin the incision in the mid portion of the hypertrophied muscle and then to extend it proximally and distally to the limits indicated.

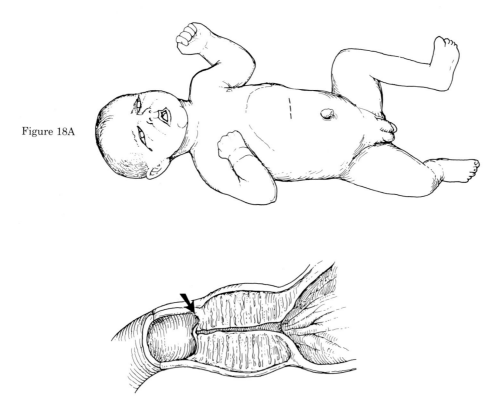

Figure 18A

Figure 18B

The initial incision should go only through the serosa and the most superficial component of the muscle layer. The hypertrophied muscle is split by blunt dissection with the handle of a knife or forceps (Fig. 18*D*). This blunt dissection reduces the likelihood of mucosal disruption.

The muscle is further separated with either the backside of a curved clamp (Fig. 18*E*), keeping the points away from the mucosa, or with a Benson pyloric spreader (Fig. 18*F*). Care should be taken not to violate the mucosa at the duodenal end. However, it is important that the distal circular muscle ring be broken. This can be determined by palpating the split in the muscle or by the mobility of the superior/inferior pyloric muscle, which will confirm that the muscle ring is no longer in continuity. On the antral end, the muscles sometimes do not divide easily with blunt dissection, and it may be necessary to divide a few residual muscle fibers sharply. Bleeding points on the serosal margins may be controlled with electrocautery, but cauterizing the exposed submucosa should be avoided.

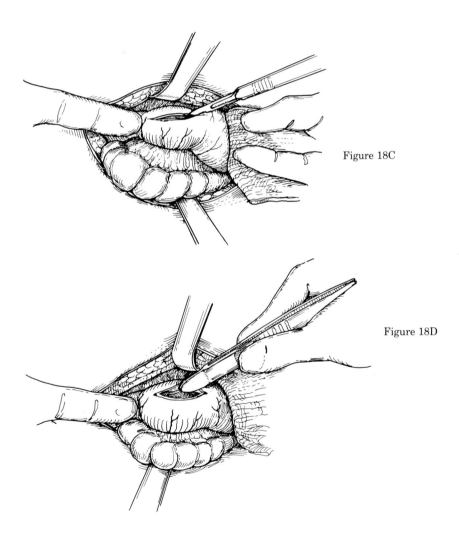

Figure 18C

Figure 18D

Figure 18*G* depicts the effect of the pyloromyotomy and how the cross-sectional area of the pylorus is increased by mucosal ballooning into the incision.

Feedings are started with clear liquids 6 to 12 hours postoperatively, increasing to full formula. Frequent burping is helpful during the postoperative period to avoid gastric distention and vomiting. The patient is usually discharged within 24 hours of the operation.

The most likely complication of pyloromyotomy is disruption of the duodenal mucosa. If the duodenum is suspected to have been entered, this can usually be confirmed by milking duodenal contents back toward the pylorus. The mucosa may be closed with inverting absorbable suture and the pyloromyotomy reapproximated. A second pyloromyotomy is then done farther superiorly. Alternatively, an omental patch is loosely approximated over the mucosal wound and feedings are withheld for 24 hours.

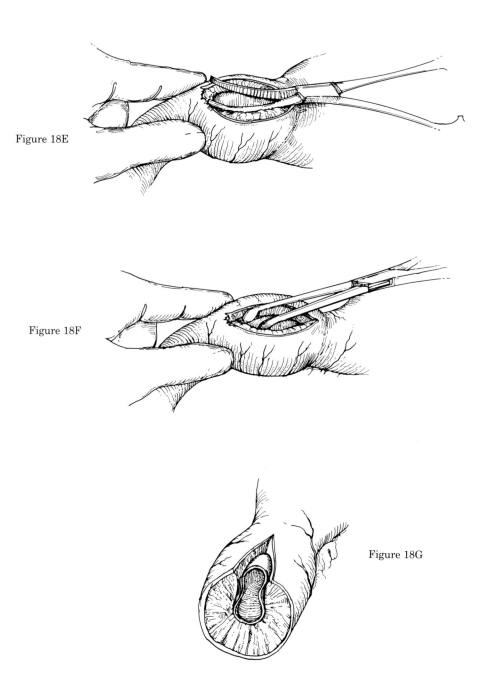

Figure 18E

Figure 18F

Figure 18G

Reference

Dudgeon DL: Lesions of the stomach. In Ashcraft KW, Holder TM, eds: Pediatric Surgery. 2nd ed. Philadelphia, WB Saunders, 1993, pp 289–304.

CHAPTER

19

Duodenal obstruction

Duodenal atresia, stenosis, and annular pancreas most often produce bilious vomiting in the newborn period and the characteristic "double-bubble" radiographic appearance with an air-fluid level in the stomach and another in the duodenum. Absence of gas beyond the duodenum suggests the diagnosis of duodenal atresia, whereas gas beyond the junction of the second and third portions of the duodenum suggests stenosis or annular pancreas. Duodenal atresia may be complete (Fig. 19A), with discontinuity in the muscular wall of the bowel. The seromuscular layers may be in continuity with the atresia, as represented by a complete membrane (Fig. 19B). An incomplete membrane may also be seen, forming a "windsock" deformity in the dilated duodenum with such a small opening that only a small proportion of the duodenal contents is passed to the distal intestine. Annular pancreas (Fig. 19C) may be associated with either complete interruption of the lumen or a high-grade partial obstruction. It is not advisable to attempt division of the pancreatic tissue surrounding the duodenum, as this may produce pancreatic leak and incompletely relieve the obstructive process.

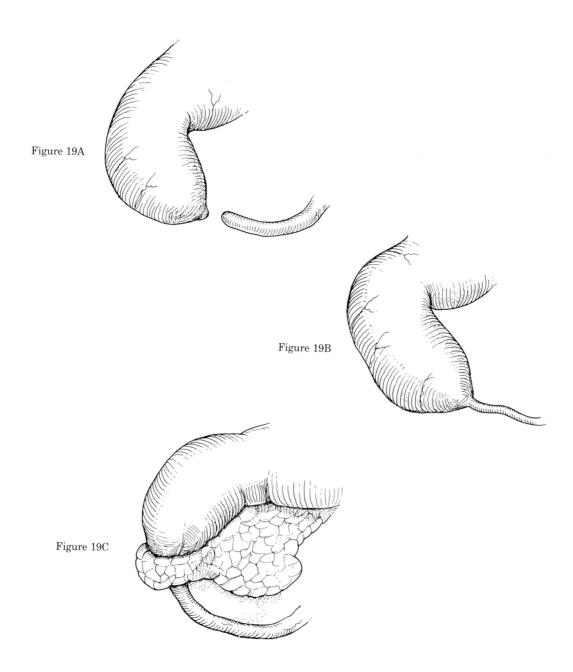

Figure 19A

Figure 19B

Figure 19C

The duodenal web or membrane very often occurs at or near the ampulla of Vater (Fig. 19D). When there is continuity of the muscular coats of the bowel, the best surgical approach is through a longitudinal incision in the dilated duodenum. The ampulla of Vater should be identified, which is sometimes aided by squeezing the gallbladder. Complete excision of the duodenal membrane is preferable while protecting the ampulla. The proximal and distal mucosal edges may be approximated by absorbable suture. Transverse closure of the longitudinal duodenotomy incision guards against further narrowing of the duodenum.

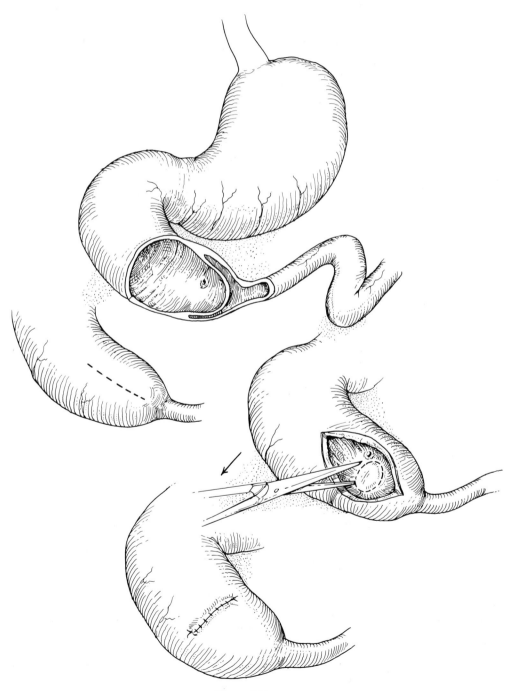

Figure 19D

In the patient with annular pancreas or complete interruption of the duodenal continuity, a duodenoduodenostomy should be accomplished. The distal duodenum is sometimes difficult to locate, although the two ends are usually in proximity (Fig. 19E). The best approach is to take down the attachments of the right colon, reflecting it medially and inferiorly to allow access (Fig. 19F).

A transverse incision is made in the proximal dilated duodenum, again attempting to locate the ampulla of Vater. The incision should not be carried far enough medially to put the ampulla at risk of injury or suture obstruction. A longitudinal incision of comparable size is then made in the distal duodenum. An anastomosis using continuous absorbable suture is made between the distal and the proximal duodenum (Fig. 19G). This same approach is used in the treatment of an annular pancreas.

The completed anastomosis is seen in Figure 19H. The colon is replaced in its original position.

The primary complication of an operative procedure to correct duodenal atresia or stenosis is delayed function of the bowel. This is due to the large diameter of the duodenum. Some surgeons have recommended plication of this portion of the intestine to improve its peristalsis. Recurrent stenosis— whether caused by formation of intraluminal adhesions after a web is excised or by anastomotic stricture—seems to be more common after correction of duodenal obstruction than after anastomosis for more distal bowel obstruction.

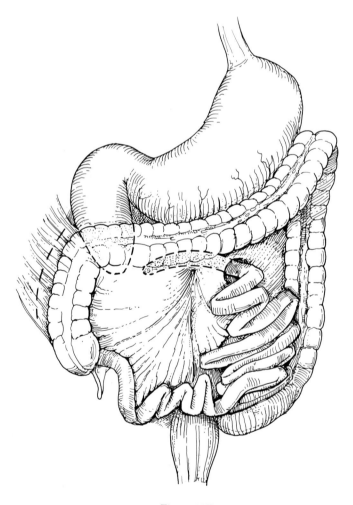

Figure 19E

Total parenteral nutrition is necessary during the 2 to 3 weeks of delayed bowel function. If obstruction persists after 3 weeks, a contrast radiographic study should be performed to determine that the anastomosis is open.

Down syndrome is commonly associated with duodenal atresia. Esophageal atresia and tracheoesophageal fistula may also be seen.

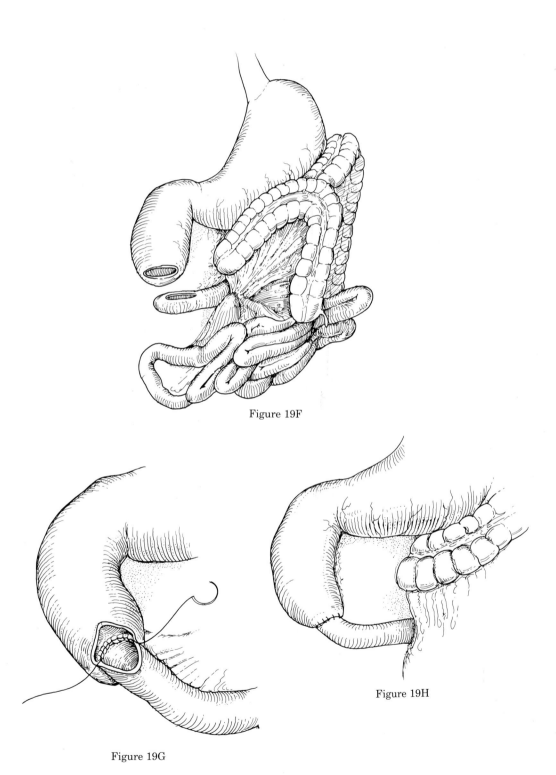

Figure 19F

Figure 19G

Figure 19H

References

Weber TR, Lewis JE, Mooney D: Duodenal atresia: a comparison of techniques of repair. J Pediatr Surg 21:1133, 1986.

Dickson JAS: Apple peel small bowel. An uncommon variant of duodenal and jejunal atresia. J Pediatr Surg 5:595, 1970.

Guttman FM, Braun P, Bensoussan AL: The pathogenesis of intestinal atresia. Surg Gynecol Obstet 141:203, 1975.

Puri P, Fujimoto T: New observations on the pathogenesis of multiple intestinal atresias. J Pediatr Surg 23:221, 1988.

CHAPTER

20

Malrotation

During fetal development, the intestine, which elongates much more than does the fetus, protrudes into the umbilical cord as a loop (Fig. 20*A*). The portion of the intestine that protrudes outside the abdominal cavity involves the mid duodenum down to approximately the splenic flexure of the colon. As the fetal abdomen enlarges, the intestine undergoes a process of counterclockwise rotation during which it is drawn back into the abdominal cavity (Fig. 20*B*). The ascending colon becomes fixed in the retroperitoneum, as does the terminal portion of the duodenum, forming a broad base for the mesentery. The fixation extends from the ligament of Treitz down to the lateral attachments of the cecum (Fig. 20*C*). Fixation of the proximal duodenum at the head of the pancreas and retroperitoneal fixation of the descending colon occur independently of this rotational process.

In patients with incomplete rotation and fixation, two processes may occur to produce intestinal obstruction. The first and most constant is the presence of bands of peritoneum that extend from the hepatic flexure and right colon across the duodenum to attach in the region of the right kidney. These bands, called Ladd's bands, compress the duodenum from the outside, producing obstruction to the passage of duodenal contents. This is an incomplete obstruction that very frequently manifests itself as vomiting in the newborn (Fig. 20*D*). Plain radiographs of the abdomen may show gas in the stomach and the first portion of the duodenum but also usually show distal bowel gas, which prevents clear identification of the disorder. Contrast radiographic studies must be used to delineate the problem. Two approaches to this have been taken. A barium enema will show that the cecum is not normally located in the right lower quadrant, but the limitation of this study is that the pressure of the barium may push the cecum into the right lower abdomen, and the suspected diagnosis of malrotation may not be clearly confirmed. A much better means of determining the presence of malrotation and duodenal obstruction is the upper gastrointestinal study with small bowel follow-through. Contrast will be seen to enter the stomach and the first portion of the duodenum; often there is a disparity in size between the first portion and the remainder of the duodenum. There may be little contrast passing into the small intestine. Additionally, no "C" loop is formed, and the ligament of Treitz

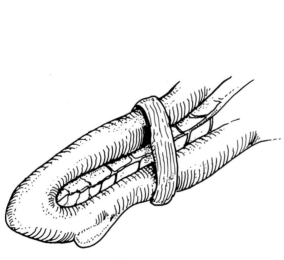

Figure 20A

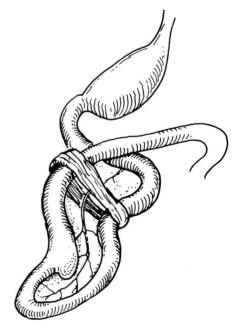

Figure 20B

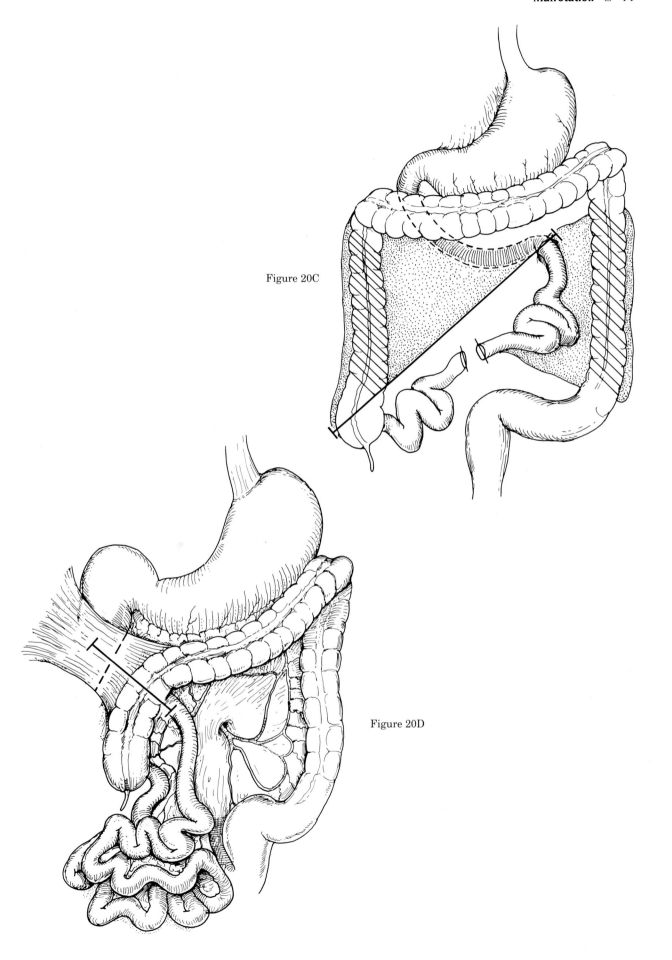

Figure 20C

Figure 20D

is nonexistent. The duodenum will fall away in a corkscrew manner to the right of the spine.

Midgut volvulus may occur when the intestine twists on the narrow mesentery, completely obstructing the lumen and compromising its own blood supply (Fig. 20E). This is the most emergent pediatric intestinal crisis that can occur, as irreversible gangrene may develop within a few hours. Although this process may occur in the newborn, it may also occur in older patients who have had little or no intestinal symptoms before the volvulus. Volvulus produces very severe, unrelenting abdominal pain, almost always associated with bilious vomiting. Marked abdominal tenderness is present. An upper gastrointestinal contrast study is usually done to confirm the disorder and will show a very tight corkscrew appearance at the mid portion of the duodenum.

Patients who show radiographic evidence of obstructive Ladd's bands or evidence of volvulus should undergo urgent operation. The operative purpose is to devolve the bowel if it is twisted and to restore circulation immediately. The area of the duodenal loop is then explored to divide Ladd's bands. Ladd's bands extend from the hepatic flexure of the colon to the right upper lateral abdominal wall; they cover the duodenum and may at first appear not to be significant. They should be divided completely so that the duodenum is no longer retroperitoneal; at this point the right colon will be completely mobile.

It has been suggested that broad-based fixation of the bowel is best attempted by placing the cecum up in the splenic flexure and suturing the cecum to the colon at that point. The appendix should be removed to prevent the development of appendicitis in a very atypical location, which could lead to disastrous consequences (Fig. 20F). Thus the new line of fixation of the mesentery extends from the porta hepatis across to the splenic flexure. This widened base theoretically should reduce the likelihood of recurrent volvulus; however, volvulus can recur after this procedure. Anecdotally, it appears that patients with malrotation and volvulus tend to form fewer adhesions than other patients, because recurrent volvulus is common. Plication of the cecum to the splenic flexure or of small bowel loops to each other often is fraught with disappointment. The sutures seem to pull loose and allow the volvulus to recur in spite of the surgeon's best efforts.

Any patient who has undergone an operation for malrotation with or without volvulus must be warned that immediate medical attention should be sought in the event of bilious vomiting.

The most disastrous complication of volvulus is irreversible gangrene of the bowel. In these patients we usually elect to untwist the bowel, place it in its normal position, close the incision, and then return 12 to 24 hours later for a second look. During this time, the parents need to be approached with regard to their wishes for additional operative intervention. It is possible to resect all of the dead bowel, leaving the patient with insufficient intestine to survive. Some parents elect to forego heroic efforts that would commit the child to a lifetime of total parenteral nutrition. The outlook for these patients may improve in the future, depending on the status of small bowel transplantation.

References

Groff, D: Malrotation. In Ashcraft KW, Holder TM, eds: Pediatric Surgery. 2nd ed. Philadelphia, WB Saunders, 1993, pp 320–330.

Filston HC, Kirks DR: Malrotation—the ubiquitous anomaly. J Pediatr Surg 16:614–620, 1981.

Powell DM, Othersen HB, Smith CD: Malrotation of the intestines in children: the effect of age on presentation and therapy. J Pediatr Surg 24:777–780, 1989.

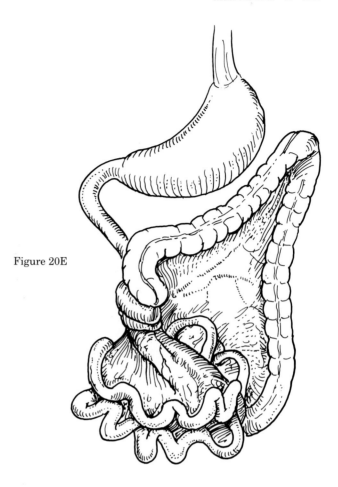

Figure 20E

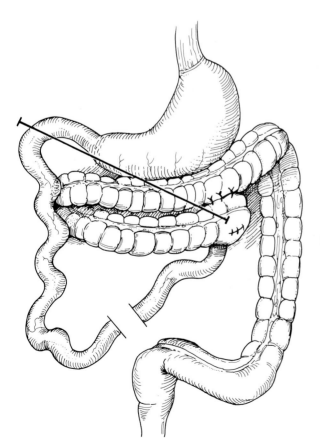

Figure 20F

21

Portoenterostomy (Kasai procedure)

Biliary atresia is a fatal disease. Most commonly all of the extrahepatic ducts are atretic (Fig. 21A), but on rare occasions there is atresia of only the distal common bile duct with a patent common hepatic duct (Fig. 21B). This is best treated by choledochojejunostomy (Roux-en-Y jejunostomy). Rarely, a hypoplastic common duct will provide communication between the gallbladder and the duodenum with atretic proximal extrahepatic ducts (Fig. 21C). When there is no proximal hepatic duct, the patient is a candidate for a portoenterostomy. Some believe primary liver transplantation is preferable to portoenterostomy, because transplantation is an easier procedure for those children who have not had a previous portoenterostomy. However, portoenterostomy currently results in enough long-term survivors to warrant its continued use as the primary procedure. Continued follow-up of both groups of patients may alter this opinion.

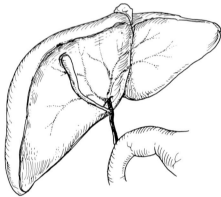

Figure 21A

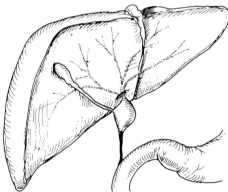

Figure 21B

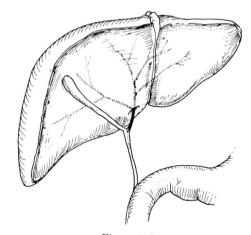

Figure 21C

The operative approach is through an upper abdominal transverse incision on the patient's right side. This incision is sufficient for the liver biopsy and cholangiogram but may easily be extended for additional exposure (Fig. 21*D*). The incision should be made just below the costal margin. In patients with a particularly large liver, this may not be the easiest approach for the Kasai procedure, but because many of these children are subsequent candidates for liver transplantation, transplantation should not be jeopardized by making the incision too low.

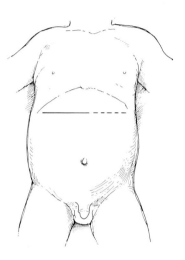

Figure 21D

The initial step of the procedure is to determine the status of the extrahepatic bile ducts by means of an operative cholangiogram through the gallbladder (Fig. 21*E*). At the time of operation, it is usually not possible to know positively whether the infant's jaundice is a result of biliary atresia or neonatal hepatitis. A small catheter is sutured into the fundus of the gallbladder with a pursestring suture, and an operative cholangiogram is obtained. If there is no filling of the proximal or distal bile ducts, the surgeon proceeds with portoenterostomy. If the duodenum fills but there is no filling of the proximal bile ducts, the cholangiogram is repeated while gentle temporary occlusion of the distal common duct is applied. This maneuver also occludes the portal vein and the hepatic artery and should be applied only during the actual repeat injection. If the repeat cholangiogram likewise fails to reveal proximal hepatic ducts, the patient should undergo portoenterostomy.

Figure 21E

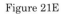
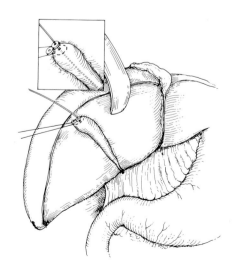

The gallbladder is dissected from the liver, and the fibrous strands of hepatic ducts are dissected proximally into the liver hilum (Fig. 21*F*). The area between the left and right portal veins is dissected free up to the area where the fibrous strand enters the liver.

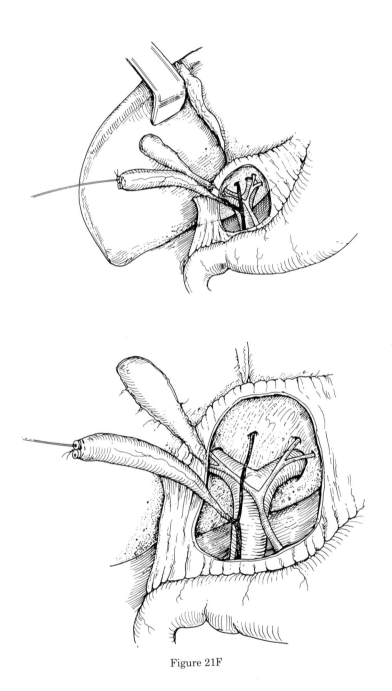

Figure 21F

The fibrous strand is then divided distally, and traction sutures are placed in the liver capsule just superior to the hepatic vessels (Fig. 21*G*).

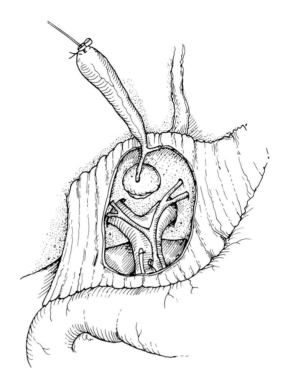

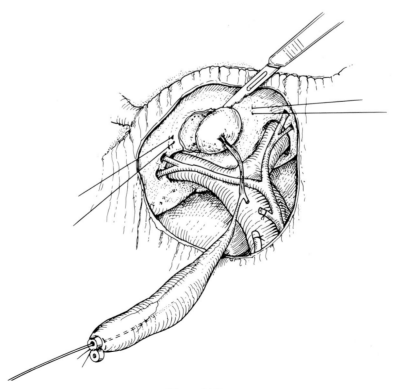

Figure 21G

A 1-cm-diameter core of capsule and liver extending 2 to 3 mm into the liver parenchyma is excised along with the fibrous tract (Fig. 21*H*). A frozen section of the liver specimen usually shows bile ducts. If these are 50 μm or more in diameter, the prognosis for a good result is better. If no ducts are detected, the core of liver is deepened another 2 to 3 mm.

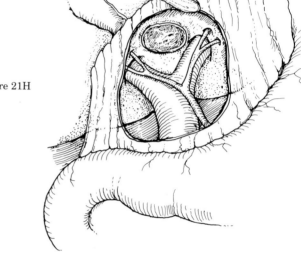

Figure 21H

The jejunum is divided at an appropriate arcade 10 to 15 cm distal to the ligament of Treitz. The distal end is then passed through the mesocolon up to the porta hepatis. The jejunum is then sutured to the liver capsule at the site of the resected button of tissue in the porta. The posterior half of the suture line is placed with interrupted sutures, which are then tied (Fig. 21*I*). The anterior half of the sutures are then likewise placed through the full thickness of the jejunum and the capsule of the liver (Fig. 21*J*).

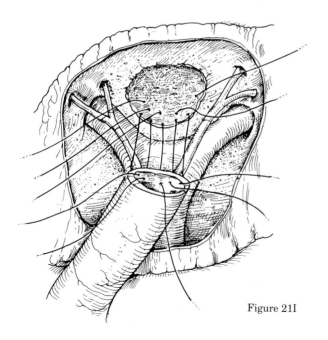

Figure 21I

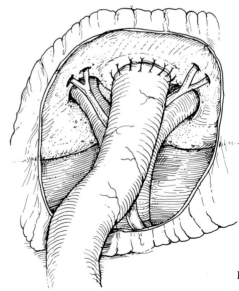

Figure 21J

The Roux-en-Y jejunostomy is then completed 30 cm below the portoenterostomy (Fig. 21*K*). The patient should be kept on broad-spectrum antibiotics for 6 weeks and on trimethoprim-sulfamethoxazole (Septra) for the first year of life.

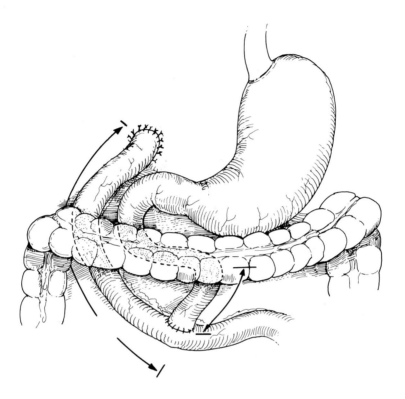

Figure 21K

Reference

Karrer FM, Lilly JR, Hall RJ: Biliary tract disorders and portal hypertension. In Ashcraft KW, Holder TM, eds: Pediatric Surgery. 2nd ed. Philadelphia, WB Saunders, 1993, pp. 478–504.

Choledochal cyst

The etiology of choledochal cyst is not definitely known, but distal common duct obstruction below the junction of the pancreatic duct with the common bile duct is very commonly seen. It is presumed that reflux of pancreatic juice into the common bile duct destroys the wall integrity and leads to cyst formation. The fact that many of these patients do not present until after infancy suggests that this is an acquired defect. Jaundice and right upper quadrant pain are the most common presentations.

Choledochal cysts are most commonly fusiform (Fig. 22A), wherein the extrahepatic common bile duct is dilated down to about the point of its entry into the pancreatic substance. There is a demonstrable narrowing of the duct below its junction with the pancreatic duct. Choledochal cysts may be saccular or may take the shape of a diverticulum off the common bile duct with a normal-appearing cystic duct and common bile duct (Fig. 22B). Less common is the choledochal cyst associated with cystic changes of the intrahepatic bile ducts (Fig. 22C).

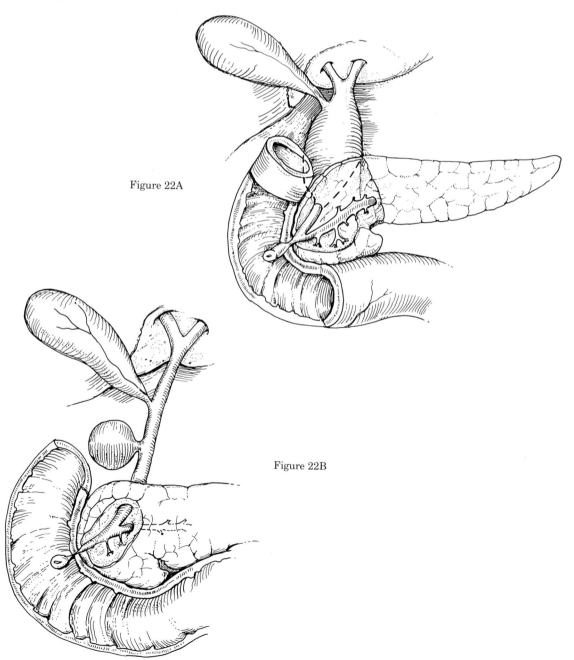

Figure 22A

Figure 22B

Caroli's disease is a very uncommon situation in which the extrahepatic bile ducts are normal, with cystic malformation only of the intrahepatic bile ducts (Fig. 22D).

Because the mucosal changes of choledochal cysts have been known to lead to malignant degeneration over time, surgical therapy is directed toward removing the abnormal mucosal lining of the dilated bile ducts. The extrahepatic bile ducts may be excised and replaced by a Roux-en-Y jejunal bile duct anastomosis. Patients with Caroli's disease may require liver transplantation for maximum protection against malignancy.

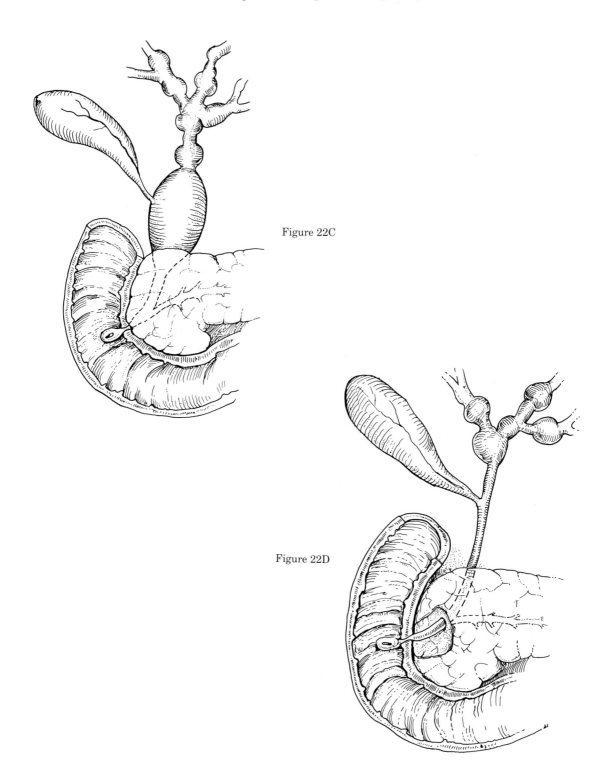

Figure 22C

Figure 22D

Thus, surgical therapy should be directed toward removing the abnormal bile ducts all the way up to the porta hepatis if necessary. Dissection downward to the juncture of the head of the pancreas will allow oversewing of the distal common bile duct. The gallbladder is removed, and the proximal ducts may be transected at the point where their diameter is near normal (Fig. 22E). Frequently the inflammatory reaction around the choledochal cyst is such that any attempt to dissect the cyst off the hepatic artery and the portal vein would be dangerous. In such instances it is best to leave the strip of fibromuscular wall of the choledochal cyst that is adherent to the portal vein and hepatic artery and to simply strip the mucosa out of that portion. The remaining free wall of the choledochal cyst is removed up to the proximal extent of the cyst. The distal end is oversewn (Fig. 22F).

A Roux-en-Y limb of jejunum is brought up in a retrocolic manner and anastomosed to the most proximal end of the bile ducts that are normal (Figs. 22G, 22H).

The most common complications occurring after this procedure are related to anastomotic stricture or anastomotic leak. Careful anastomosis of the jejunal mucosa to the mucosa of the proximal biliary tree is important.

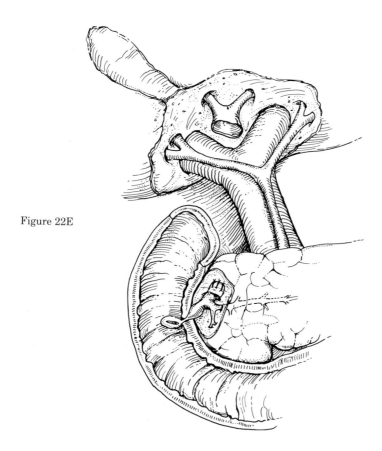

Figure 22E

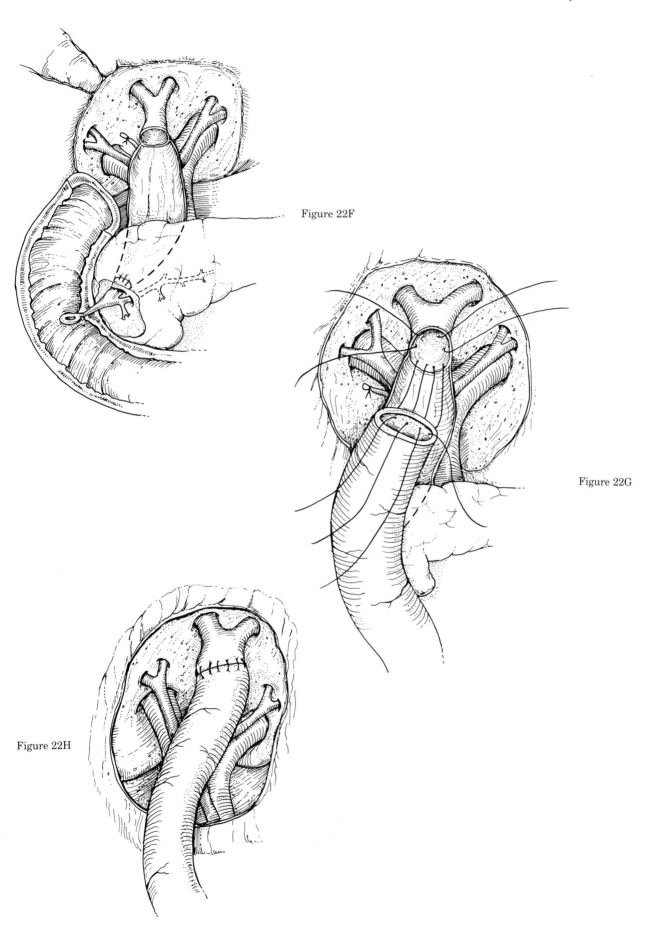

Figure 22F

Figure 22G

Figure 22H

Reference

Karrer FM, Lilly JR, Hall RJ: Biliary tract disorders and portal hypertension. In Ashcraft KW, Holder TM, eds: Pediatric Surgery. 2nd ed. Philadelphia, WB Saunders, 1993, pp 478–504.

23

Splenectomy

Elective splenectomy is done after appropriate immunization against *Pneumococcus* spp. and influenza. The patient is placed on the right side and rolled posteriorly 15 degrees. The body is flexed over a kidney rest or a rolled towel placed under the short ribs (Fig. 23*A*). A transverse incision is made just below the tip of the twelfth rib anteriorly as far as necessary to extract the spleen. Often it is possible to remove the spleen by an incision ending well lateral to the rectus muscles. On other occasions, however, the spleen is so large that it is necessary to extend the incision into the rectus or even across the midline. Usually it is possible to avoid the lower intercostal nerves by reflecting them superiorly or inferiorly.

On entering the peritoneum, the lower pole of the spleen is delivered into the wound so that it can be retracted inferiorly and anteriorly. An incision is then made in the posterior peritoneal attachment of the spleen.

Incision of the lateral splenic attachment is extended up to the superior pole (Fig. 23*B*). Using blunt dissection, the posterior and superior aspects of the spleen are freed, allowing the entire spleen to be delivered onto the abdominal wall. The intestines fall away to the right, presenting no problem in the exposure. The stomach is decompressed using a nasogastric tube, and the lesser sac is entered. The short gastric vessels are clamped and divided. The gastric end of the short gastric vessels are suture ligated, incorporating a bit of the serosa of the stomach to prevent postoperative gastric distention from dislodging a ligature (Fig. 23*C*).

The splenic artery and vein are then dissected free along the superior aspect of the tail of the pancreas. The artery and then the splenic vein are doubly ligated and divided (Fig. 23*D*). Any remaining peritoneal attachments are then divided, being careful to secure hemostasis when dividing the small veins along the superior aspect of the pancreas. A regional search for accessory spleens should be made and any residual bleeding points controlled. The nasogastric tube is then removed, and feeding is started on the first postoperative day.

If the splenectomy is being carried out for trauma or concomitant biliary procedures are to be performed, the procedure should be done with the patient supine, using either a transverse or a vertical incision. The exposure may be a little more difficult under these circumstances, but the dissection should follow the steps just described.

The major immediate complication is hemorrhage from the splenic artery or vein. Long-term complications include acute overwhelming sepsis, which may be prevented by presplenectomy immunization and the use of prophylactic antibiotics.

Reference

Ein SH: Splenic lesions. In Ashcraft KW, Holder TM, eds: Pediatric Surgery. 2nd ed. Philadelphia, WB Saunders, 1993, pp 535–545.

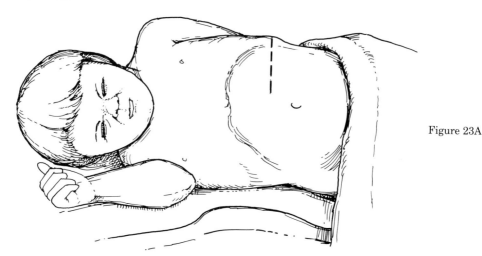

Figure 23A

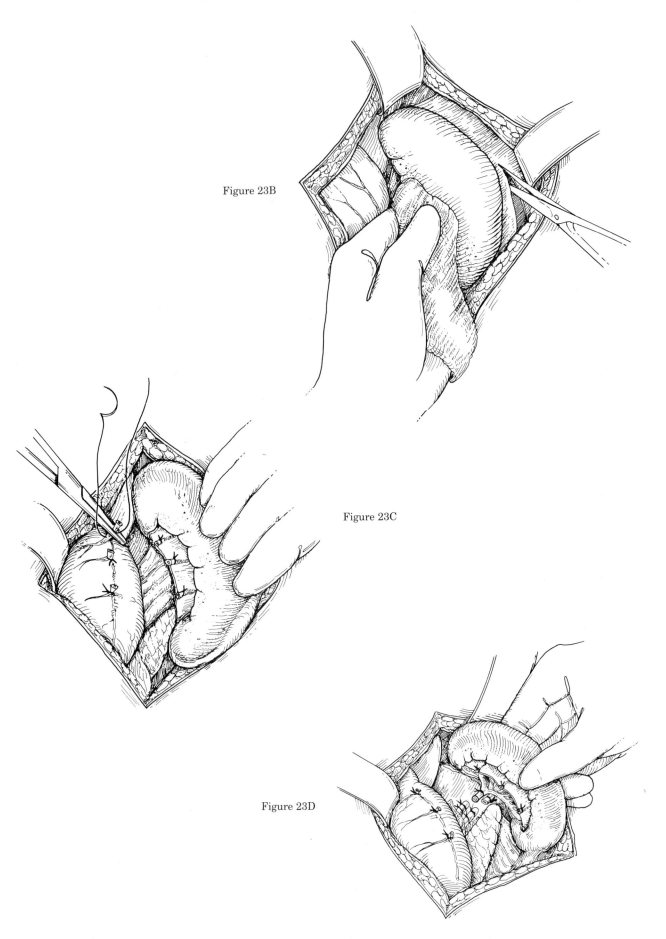

Figure 23B

Figure 23C

Figure 23D

Subtotal and total pancreatectomy

Pancreatectomy in pediatric patients is usually done for treatment of hyperinsulinism. Other indications include malignancy and trauma.

The arterial blood supply to the head of the pancreas comes from the anterior and posterior pancreaticoduodenal arteries, which also supply the "C" loop of the duodenum; the body and tail are supplied by branches from the splenic artery (Fig. 24A). Venous drainage is to the portal system. Of note are the numerous small, short, delicate vessels along the superior aspect of the body and tail of the pancreas that drain to the splenic vein.

The ductal structure within the pancreas may consist of a single duct combining with the common bile duct to join the duodenum through the ampulla of Vater. There may be an accessory pancreatic duct entering the duodenum separately and more proximally; this is known as the duct of Wirsung (Fig. 24B).

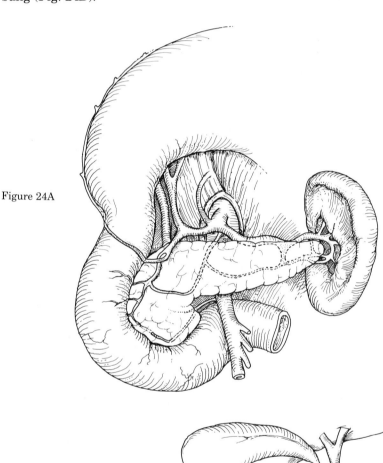

Figure 24A

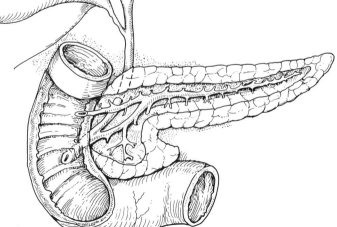

Figure 24B

DISTAL PANCREATECTOMY

Distal pancreatectomy performed either for an adenoma of the body or tail or to correct trauma-related injury is the easiest of the partial pancreatectomies and consists of removing the portion of the pancreas to the left of the "surgical neck" at the point where the pancreas crosses the aorta and superior mesenteric vessels (Fig. 24C). The vessels to the splenic vein are the most troublesome and must be individually controlled by ligature. Ligation is more secure and is less likely to cause splenic vein thrombosis than is the use of the cautery. The pancreas is transected at the level of the neck. The pancreatic duct(s) is (are) individually ligated and the neck of the pancreas transected. The anterior and posterior capsules of the pancreas (a structure more evident in name than in fact) may be approximated over the transected portion of the pancreas.

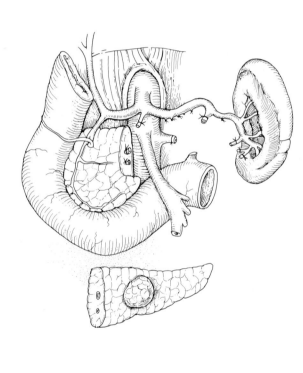

Figure 24C

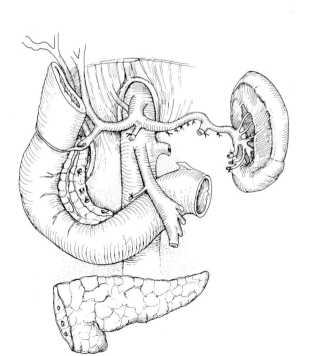

Figure 24D

SUBTOTAL PANCREATECTOMY

Subtotal pancreatectomy as treatment for nesidioblastosis requires removal of 85% to 95% of the pancreas (i.e., the tail, body, and most of the head of the pancreas) (Fig. 24D). The two areas of concern are injury to the common bile duct as it passes through the head of the pancreas on its way to the duodenum and devascularization of a portion of the duodenum by resection of the pancreaticoduodenal vessels.

Dissection begins with mobilization of the distal pancreas and proceeds to the right. The uncinate process is identified and its blood supply divided. The head of the pancreas is dissected off the duodenum inferiorly to the inferior portion of the C loop. Superiorly, the dissection is carried along toward the hepatic artery. The common bile duct should be followed to the point where it enters the head of the pancreas. A crescent-shaped portion of the head of the pancreas remains on the inner surface of the duodenum, preserving the pancreaticoduodenal vessels and the common bile duct. Individual vessels and ducts on the cut surface are ligated. Close attention must be paid to the patient's serum glucose and insulin levels during the postoperative period.

In children, it is occasionally necessary to perform a pancreatectomy (Fig. 24E) or to remove the head of the pancreas for treatment of malignant disease or trauma (Fig. 24F). Removal of the head of the pancreas requires removal of the duodenum. In addition to the distal dissection described previously, it is necessary to mobilize the duodenum and determine that there is no contraindication to this radical procedure (i.e., involvement of the portal vein by spread of tumor). The duodenum is reflected medially by making an incision in the peritoneum to the right of the duodenum. The common bile duct and portal vein are identified and dissected free superior to the duodenum; then, using blunt and sharp dissection, the portal vein is dissected free from the head of the pancreas to determine resectability. The stomach is divided proximal to the antrum, and the antrum and pylorus are removed with the specimen. The common bile duct is divided superior to the pancreas. The pancreas is then freed from the portal and superior mesenteric vessels, and the jejunum is transected beyond the ligament of Treitz. Thus, the pancreas, duodenum, and distal common bile duct are removed en bloc. The continuity of the intestinal tract and biliary drainage are accomplished by closing over the end of the jejunum. The common bile duct is sutured into the proximal jejunum using circumferential through-and-through sutures and then sutured into the side of the proximal residual jejunum. The gastrojejunostomy completes the procedure (Fig. 24E).

The distal portion of the pancreas, if preserved, can be placed into the proximal end of the jejunum. The pancreatic duct is left to drain into the proximal jejunum, which is sutured to the pancreatic capsule with permanent sutures (Fig. 24F).

COMPLICATIONS

The most serious complication of a distal pancreatectomy or of subtotal pancreatectomy in which the head and body are removed (Whipple procedure) is a pancreatic leak. After all pancreatic procedures, the area should be drained.

The most serious complication of a subtotal distal pancreatectomy is injury to the duodenum or the common bile duct. Extreme caution must be exercised during transection of the proximal pancreas. It is better to leave too much residual pancreas in the C loop than to risk devascularization of the duodenum.

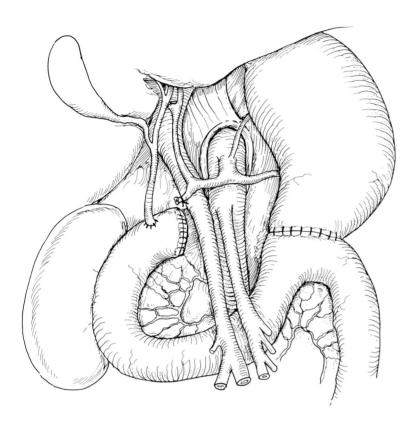

Figure 24E

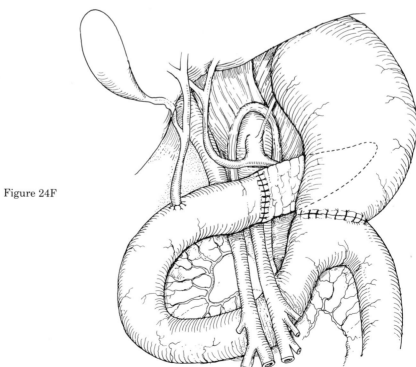

Figure 24F

Reference

Vane DW: Lesions of the pancreas. In Ashcraft KW, Holder TM, eds: Pediatric Surgery. 2nd ed. Philadelphia, WB Saunders, 1993, pp 525–534.

Splenorenal shunt

Bleeding from esophageal varices is a result of obstruction of flow through the portal vein and liver. Natural collaterals develop to decompress the portal bed. These can occur through the hemorrhoidal veins, the round ligament, and the submucosal esophageal venous plexus (Fig. 25A). Collaterals to the esophagus are by way of the splenic vein, the short gastric veins into the submucosal veins of the fundus, and the coronary vein from the portal vein. Avoidance of aspirin or similar medications in patients with portal hypertension has greatly reduced the incidence of variceal bleeding. Currently the treatment of choice for bleeding esophageal varices is endoscopic sclerotherapy or rubber-band ligation, either of which is usually successful. Because of complications, an occasional child is a candidate for a decompression shunting procedure.

The etiology of portal hypertension in children is most often thrombosis with cavernous transformation of the portal vein. Umbilical vein catheterization has been implicated as one of the most common predisposing factors. After about two decades during which umbilical vein catheters were strictly avoided, their use is now on the increase. Intrahepatic blockage (i.e., with a normal portal vein) may result from biliary cirrhosis secondary to biliary atresia, cystic fibrosis, or other significant forms of intrahepatic liver disease such as congenital hepatic fibrosis. Those patients with severe intrahepatic disease are probably best treated by liver transplantation.

The most desirable form of portal decompression is a splenorenal shunt. This is most often successful when the vessels are 1 cm or more in diameter, as there has been a disappointing incidence of thrombosis in shunts less than this size. Splenic and renal veins of 1 cm or more are most often seen in children weighing more than 50 pounds. The distal splenorenal shunt is the shunt of choice (Fig. 25B), as it does not require the removal of the spleen. This shunt successfully decompresses the spleen and usually alleviates hypersplenism secondary to portal venous obstruction.

The splenorenal shunt is carried out through a left upper quadrant transverse excision extending into the flank. First the left renal vein is isolated. This vein is longer than the right and usually is an adequate vessel for a shunt. The splenic vein is dissected along the superior aspect of the pancreas, preserving its tributaries to the stomach. It is divided at its union with the inferior mesenteric vein, and the proximal end is oversewn. The splenic end is temporarily but gently occluded, as is the renal vein near the vena cava and the kidney. The divided distal end of the splenic vein is then sutured to the top of the renal vein, from which a small ellipse of appropriate size has been excised. Two corner stitches are placed using 6-0 or 7-0 Gore-Tex or Prolene sutures. The back row of the anastomosis is made from the inside using a continuous suture, being careful not to pursestring the suture line. Likewise, the anterior anastomosis is placed with continuous permanent suture interrupted in one or two places to allow growth.

The proximal splenorenal shunt is similar to the distal, except that the splenic vein is divided near the hilum of the spleen and used for the anastomosis (Fig. 25B, inset). This procedure does not decompress the spleen and may lead to continued hypersplenism or may necessitate splenectomy. In either case, the coronary vein is divided.

The side-to-side splenorenal shunt procedure combines the best of both procedures but is technically more difficult (Fig. 25C).

Thrombosis of the shunt is a serious complication. Low pressure and low flow of this venous shunt makes careful suture technique and gentle handling of these veins most important.

Reference

Altman RP, Krug J: Portal hypertension: American Academy of Pediatrics, Surgical Section Survey. J Pediatr Surg 17:567, 1982.

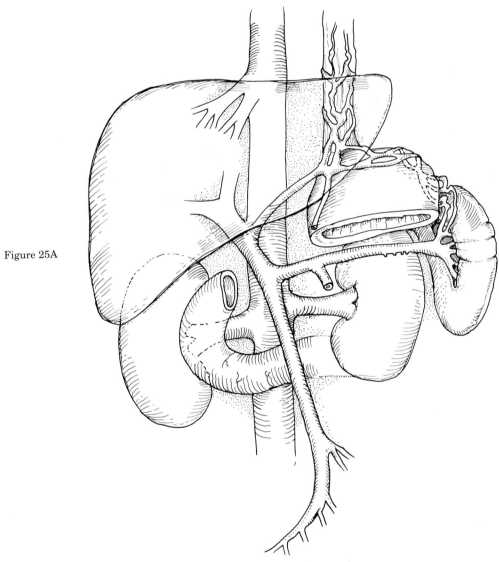

Figure 25A

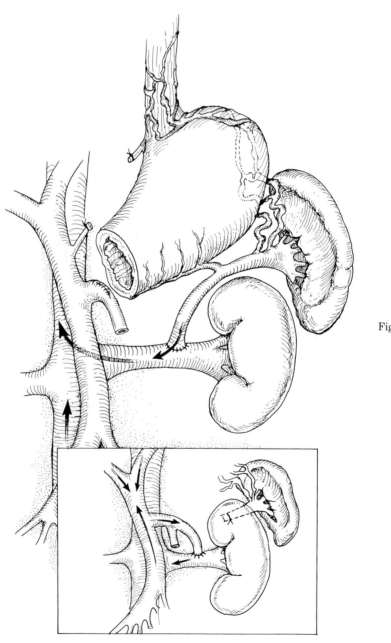

Figure 25B

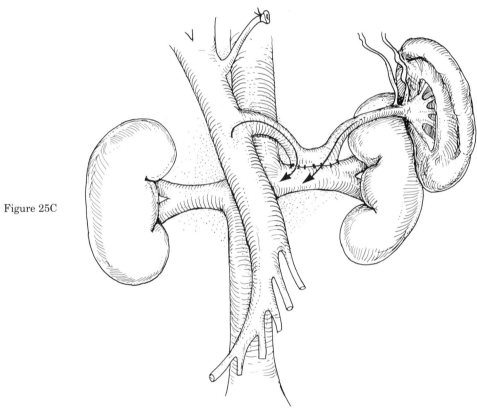

Figure 25C

Mesocaval and portocaval shunt

A patient who is not a candidate for a splenorenal shunt because of size, previous splenectomy, or other factors and who does not have a suitable portal vein because of previous thrombosis may be a candidate for a mesocaval shunt. There are two types of mesocaval shunts. The procedure proposed by Clatworthy and Boles utilizes division of the infrarenal vena cava. The distal end is oversewn and the proximal end sutured to the side of the superior mesenteric vein as cephalad as possible (Fig. 26A). The mesentery is usually thick and quite vascular, and this can be a difficult procedure. In this procedure, no prosthetic material is used. An iliac vein branch may be used for this shunt to preserve the continuity of the vena cava. The leg or legs develop collateral to the paravertebral veins, but edema is frequently present.

The other mesocaval shunt (Drapanas) utilizes a prosthetic graft to join the mesenteric vein with the inferior vena cava (Fig. 26B). This procedure is useful in larger children and adults. As the prosthesis does not grow, it is of limited value in small children.

Portocaval shunts are of limited value in children, because the portal vein is frequently thrombosed and is not suitable for a shunt. Biliary atresia, cystic fibrosis, and idiopathic hepatic fibrosis produce venous intrahepatic obstruction. Patients with this form of portal hypertension are candidates for a portocaval shunt. The side-to-side portocaval shunt is preferable, as it allows for decompression of the liver and of the portal bed (Fig. 26C).

An upper abdominal transverse incision extending into the flanks allows adequate exposure. The liver is retracted superiorly, and an incision is made in the peritoneum lateral to the duodenum (Fig. 26D, upper inset), which is reflected medially (Fig. 26D). The common bile duct and hepatic artery are dissected off the portal vein and reflected toward the midline. The portal vein is then dissected proximally and distally as required to supply sufficient mobilization for side-to-side approximation. This may require entrance into the lesser sac to free the splenic and mesenteric veins sufficiently for mobilization (Fig. 26D, lower inset). Clamps are applied on the vena cava and portal vein proximally and distally. Opposing incisions are made in the anterior aspect of the vena cava and the posterior aspect of the portal vein; 6-0 or 7-0 permanent or monofilament absorbable sutures are used for the anastomosis. The posterior suture line is constructed from the inside using a continuous suture. This suture is then continued along the anterior aspect to complete the anastomosis, taking care to avoid pursestringing (Figs. 26E, 26F).

On occasion, the anatomy precludes a side-to-side portocaval shunt, and an end-to-side shunt is employed (Fig. 26G). The portal vein is transected, the hepatic end sewn over, and the proximal end sutured into the anterior aspect of the nearby inferior vena cava. The suture technique is the same as that described for the side-to-side portocaval anastomosis. The disadvantage of this shunt is that it does not decompress the liver.

The most likely early complication of the shunt procedures is ammonia intoxication, although the distal splenorenal shunt is least likely to be associated with this complication. Thrombosis with recurrent portal hypertension may be seen. Hypersplenism, if persistent, may necessitate splenectomy with its attendant risks.

References

Clatworthy HW, Boles ET: Extrahepatic portal bed block in children: pathogenesis and treatment. Ann Surg 150:371, 1959.
Drapanas T: Interposition mesocaval shunt for treatment of portal hypertension. Ann Surg 176:435, 1972.

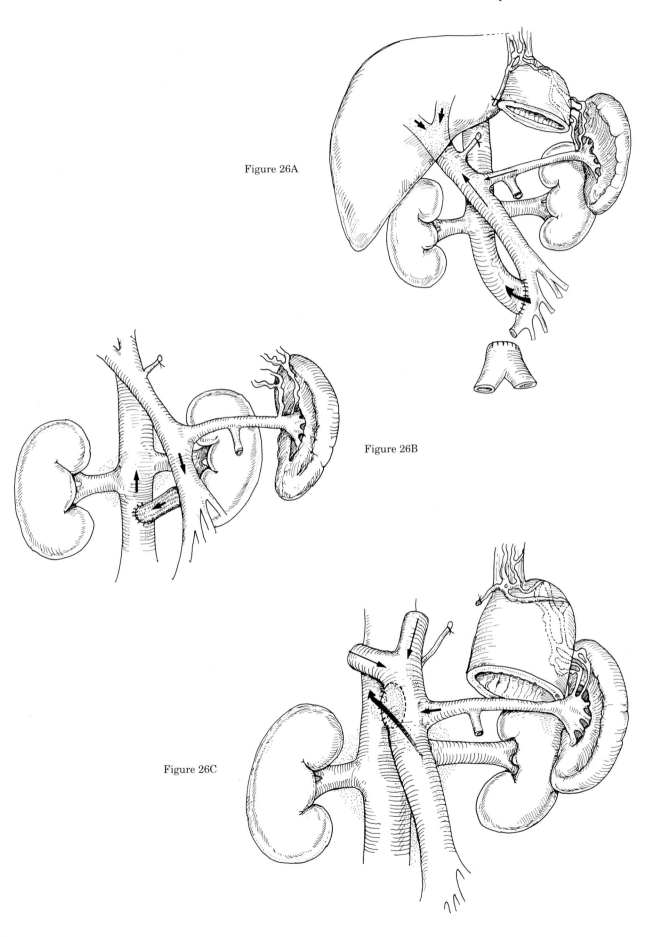

Figure 26A

Figure 26B

Figure 26C

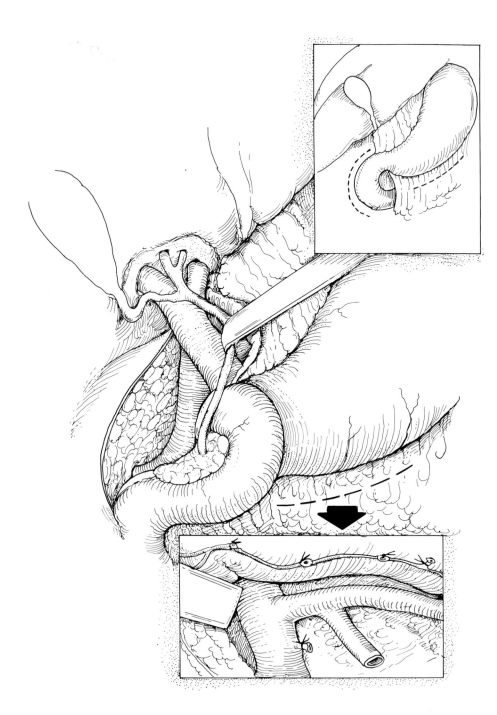

Figure 26D

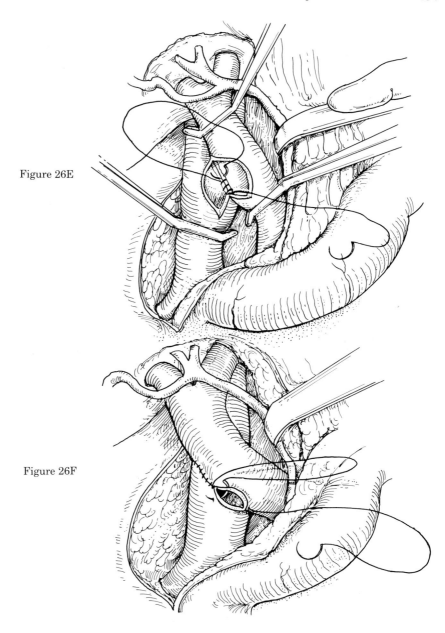

Figure 26E

Figure 26F

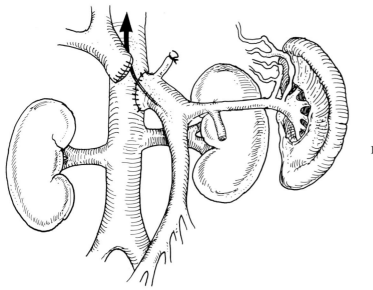

Figure 26G

CHAPTER

27

Intestinal atresia

Intestinal atresia is the result of an in utero vascular accident and may take a number of forms. Most commonly there is no continuity of the bowel, and a gap exists in the mesentery (Fig. 27A). There are usually marked dilatation and hypertrophy of the proximal gut. The amount of missing bowel is difficult to estimate.

The lumen may be atretic while the muscular wall remains intact. The mesentery is also intact. The bowel is of normal length (Fig. 27B), and there is dilatation of the bowel proximal to the atresia. There may be multiple areas of atresia in this type, as in other types in which disparity of bowel size is seen only proximal to the first atretic area.

Atresias may be multiple with multiple mesenteric gaps (Fig. 27C). Serious loss of bowel length is usual in these patients.

One of the most difficult forms of intestinal atresia involves the blood supply to the distal segment from the right colic or ileocolic vessels. This is known as a "Christmas tree" deformity because of the appearance of the distal intestine wrapped around its vascular trunk (Fig. 27D). In all forms of atresia, the bowel distal to the atresia is small because of lack of use. However, it has the potential to function normally once the continuity in the intestinal tract has been re-established.

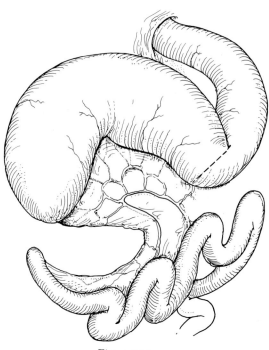

Figure 27A

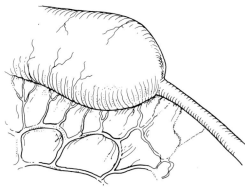

Figure 27B

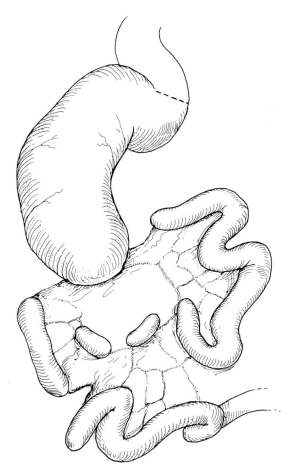

Figure 27C

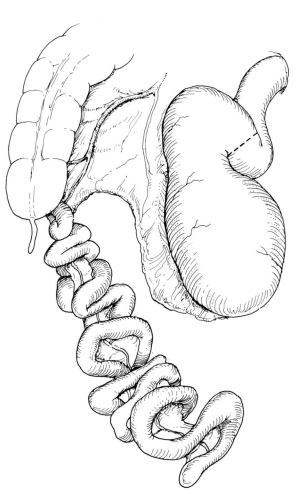

Figure 27D

An end-to-end or end-to-back anastomosis should be done between bowel ends of different size. The first step is to determine the continuity of the distal segment. This is accomplished by injection of sterile mineral oil or sterile saline into the distal bowel lumen (Fig. 27E). The contents are then "milked" through the distal bowel to ensure that the lumen is patent to the cecum. The bulbous proximal end (usually 10 to 15 cm) does not empty well, because the bowel wall does not coapt. If there is adequate length of gut, this segment should be resected. If every centimeter must be preserved, plication of this portion may be effective in improving peristalsis.

The end of the distal segment is excised and an incision made down the antimesenteric border; the length of this incision should equal the circumference of the proximal gut at the chosen line of anastomosis (Fig. 27F). Our current preference for anastomosis is a two-layer continuous suture using 6-0 or 7-0 polydioxanone, which is a monofilament, slowly absorbed suture.

The continuous suture technique is accomplished by first approximating the posterior portion of the anastomosis with full-thickness continuous locking suture (Fig. 27G). Locking suture is used so that the suture line will not be shortened. The same locking suture continues on the anterior aspect of the anastomosis. The final few sutures are Connell sutures, which are placed and tied on the outside. The second suture layer, also a continuous locking suture, reinforces the first suture line and should use only a minimal amount of tissue.

An alternative anastomotic technique consists of interrupted, inverted, horizontal mattress sutures of 5-0 silk. These sutures are full thickness, taking a minimal amount of tissue, and are placed from and tied on the inside. Most of the anterior wall can be placed from the inside as well. The final few sutures are placed from the outside and are full-thickness bites (Fig. 27H).

After either type of anastomosis, the mesenteric defect is closed with interrupted sutures, taking care to avoid damaging the blood supply (Fig. 27I).

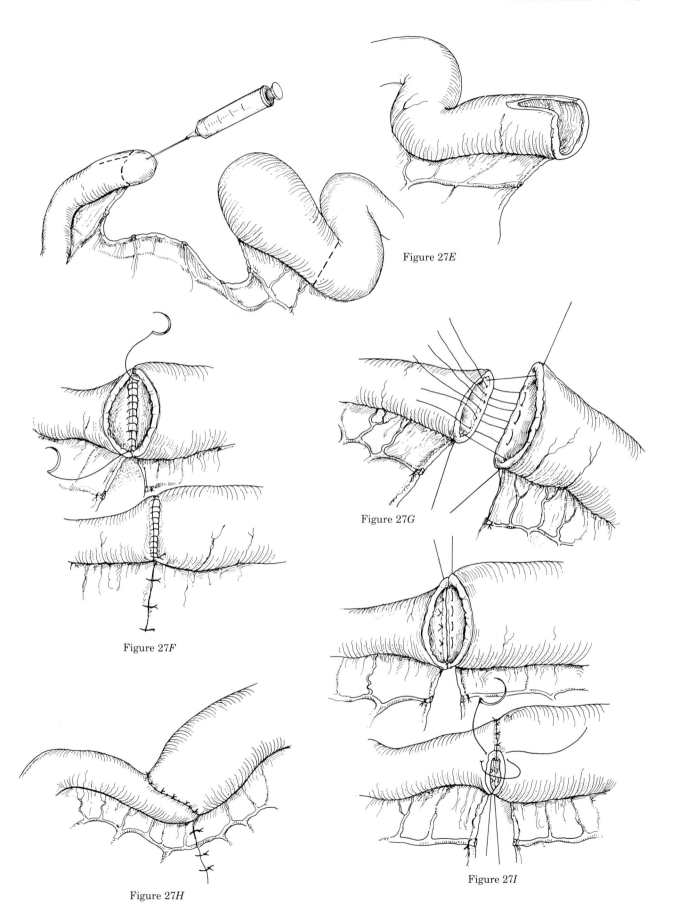

Figure 27E

Figure 27F

Figure 27G

Figure 27H

Figure 27I

The interrupted, inverted, horizontal mattress sutures provide an anastomosis of maximum diameter. The actual anastomosis requires a little more operative time. Its major disadvantage is that on rare occasions, the inverted edges have grown together, creating an anastomotic stricture requiring a second operation. We have not yet encountered this complication with the continuous locking suture technique.

The multiple atresia depicted in Figure 27C is shown repaired in Figure 27J. If there is adequate intestine, the "sausage links" may be resected and one or two anastomoses created. However, if there is a need to preserve most of the intestine, as in the figure, the bulbous tip is retained, and only the two very small segments of atretic bowel are removed. If there is sufficient length of gut, the bulbous dilated proximal segment is removed to the dashed line. Plication of the proximal dilated segment is sometimes done to reduce its diameter so that its walls can coapt when peristalsis occurs.

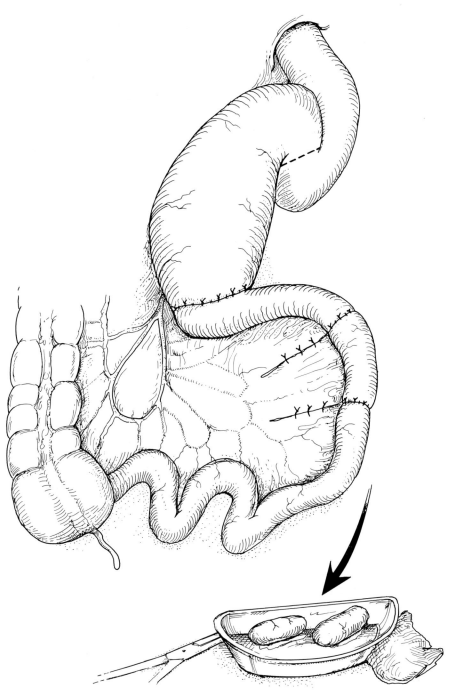

Figure 27*J*

Correction of the Christmas tree deformity is difficult (Fig. 27K). The blood supply to the end of the distal segment is often tenuous, and yet it is best to preserve all the gut possible. Unless length is a consideration, it is desirable to resect the proximal dilated segment to the dashed line in the figure. In the scenario depicted, the luminal continuity of the distal segment had been proved and all of the segment retained. Plication of the bulbous proximal gut, which is done by folding in the antimesenteric wall of the dilated gut with a series of interrupted sutures, should be considered.

Return of bowel function can sometimes be delayed several weeks. Total parenteral nutrition delivered by peripheral or central vein makes survival possible until bowel function is sufficient to maintain nutrition.

In the immediate postoperative period after correction of intestinal atresia, the major complication is an anastomotic stenosis or adhesive obstruction. It is difficult to differentiate either of these two complications from the usual long delay in return of peristalsis. This is particularly true when the bulbous proximal bowel has been retained because of bowel length concerns. After 3 weeks, a contrast study may be necessary.

Postoperative necrotizing enterocolitis (NEC) may also be seen. These episodes require cessation of oral intake, resumption of nasogastric drainage, and parenteral antibiotics (see Chapter 29).

The major long-term complication is the short-gut syndrome. It is best to support these infants with parenteral nutrition. Oral feedings are started with breast milk or predigested formula diluted to one-fourth strength. The volume of feeding is gradually increased to normal—that is, the amount of full-strength formula or milk that will provide adequate calories. The concentration of the feeding is then gradually increased. Even with adequate length of gut, this process may take up to 2 weeks to complete. Patients with insufficient length of bowel may take months or years to adapt and must be supported with central venous total parenteral nutrition.

References

Dickson JAS: Apple peel small bowel. An uncommon variant of duodenal and jejunal atresia. J Pediatr Surg 5:595, 1970.

Guttman FM, Braun P, Bensoussan AL: The pathogenesis of intestinal atresia. Surg Gynecol Obstet 141:203, 1975.

Puri P, Fujimoto T: New observations on the pathogenesis of multiple intestinal atresias. J Pediatr Surg 23:221, 1988.

Weber TR, Lewis JE, Mooney D: Duodenal atresia: a comparison of techniques of repair. J Pediatr Surg 21:1133, 1986.

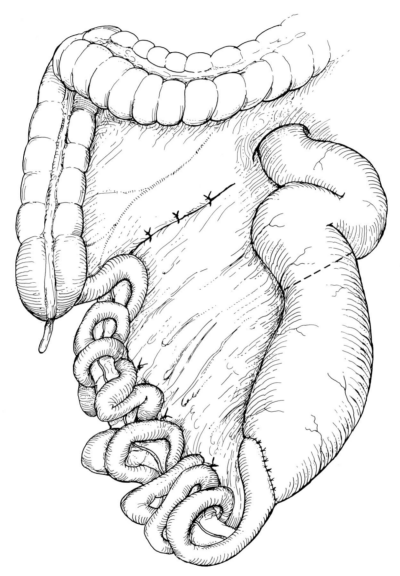

Figure 27K

28

Meconium ileus

Meconium ileus is one of the causes of neonatal intestinal obstruction and is almost always associated with cystic fibrosis. The lack of pancreatic enzymes results in the formation of a mass of inordinately sticky, tenacious meconium in the mid ileum. The obstruction produces proximal dilatation of the gut. The distal ileum and often the colon are filled with small gray bits of mucus and sloughed mucosa (Fig. 28A). There is nothing inherently wrong with the motor activity of the intestine, but the meconium is too viscous to be propelled along the intestinal tract. The bulbous portion of intestine may undergo in utero volvulus, resulting in intestinal atresia or meconium peritonitis with or without pseudocyst formation.

Although diatrizoate meglumine (Gastrografin) enemas refluxed to the level of the meconium mass have been successful, most patients with meconium ileus undergo operative therapy. The problem at operation is to evacuate the sticky meconium causing the obstruction. The most direct way to do this is to resect the portion of intestine containing the obstructing meconium (Fig. 28B). Originally this was done without primary anastomosis. The first successful approach constructed a Mikulicz ileostomy in which the proximal and distal segments were sutured together along their antimesenteric border and both brought out as a double stoma (Fig. 28C). The two segments were anastomosed with a spur-crushing clamp. After the return of bowel function, extraperitoneal closure of the stomas was done. Although successful, this procedure was fraught with problems, including the blind loop syndrome.

Bishop and Koop modified this approach by resecting the most dilated ileum. They then performed a proximal end-to-distal side anastomosis with a decompression ileostomy (Fig. 28D). This allowed for extraperitoneal closure of a single stoma once bowel function returned. Intestinal transit is aided by irrigation with mucolytic enzymes instilled into the stoma.

Santulli further modified this by bringing the proximal segment out as a stoma and performing an end-to-side anastomosis using the distal segment (Fig. 28E). Both of these "chimney" procedures take advantage of the benefits of an anastomosis but at the same time provide a vent if there is distal obstruction. (See Chapter 27 for details of anastomosis and Chapter 29 for stoma formation.)

Some surgeons prefer enterotomy with evacuation of some of the inspissated meconium, followed by insertion of a T tube, which is brought out through a stab incision for postoperative irrigation with mucolytic enzyme (Fig. 28F and G). Once the function of the gut has been established, feedings are started and the T tube removed.

Our preference, based on 30 years of experience, is to remove the meconium obstruction by operative irrigation using a 2% solution of n-acetylcysteine (Mucomyst). A pursestring suture is placed in the mid portion of the dilated segment, through which is inserted a No. 20 French Robinson catheter (Fig. 28H). The disadvantages of this technique are that it is messy and very time consuming. With patience, all of the inspissated meconium can be removed through the catheter, as can the more liquid proximal meconium. The mucolytic enzyme that escapes distally allows passage of the small pellets of mucus through the anus. The enterotomy is then closed. The patient is given 2% n-acetylcysteine enemas during the postoperative period. When the gastric aspirate decreases, feedings are started. Oral enzymes are used to substitute for the pancreatic deficiency.

Five percent of patients with meconium ileus do not have an abnormal result on sweat test—the indicator of the presence of cystic fibrosis. The infant will not produce enough sweat in the first month of life to make a sweat test possible, so it may be a month or more before the question of cystic fibrosis is resolved.

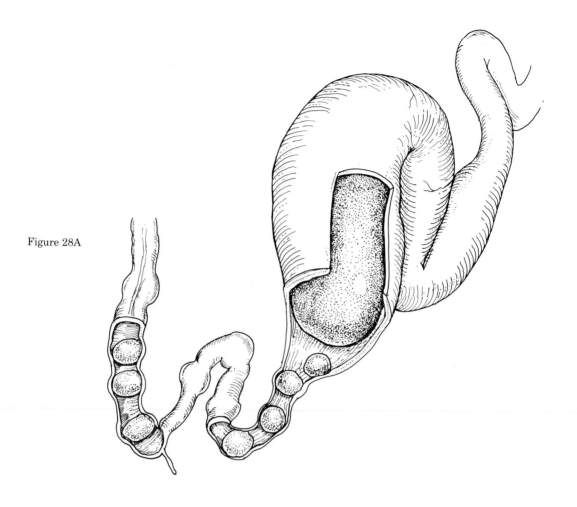

Figure 28A

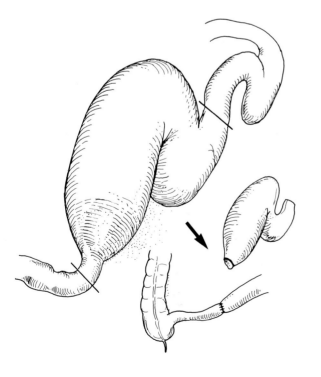

Figure 28B

The early postoperative complications concern the return of peristalsis to the dilated ileum. Patience, adequate parenteral nutrition, and *n*-acetylcysteine enemas are important. The late complications center on the underlying respiratory disorder, cystic fibrosis.

References

Bishop HC, Koop CE: Management of meconium ileus: resection, roux-en Y anastomosis and ileostomy irrigation with pancreatic enzymes. Ann Surg 145:410–414, 1957.
Santulli TV, Blanc WA: Congenital atresia of the intestine: pathogenesis and treatment. Ann Surg 154:939–948, 1961.

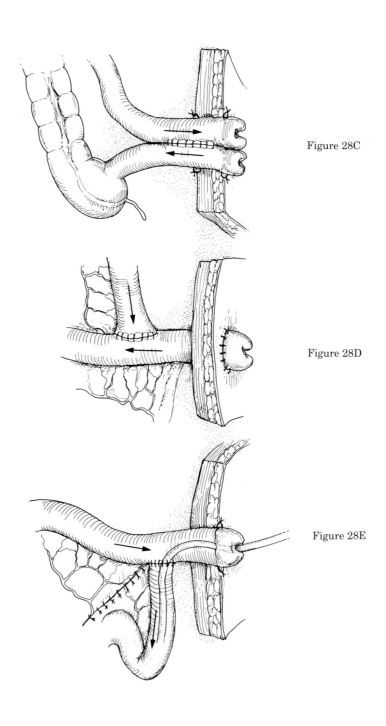

Figure 28C

Figure 28D

Figure 28E

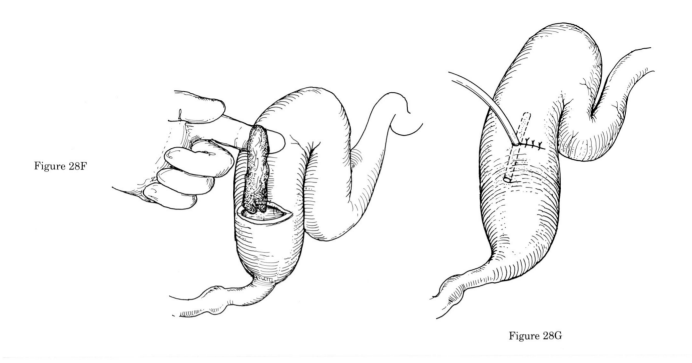

Figure 28F

Figure 28G

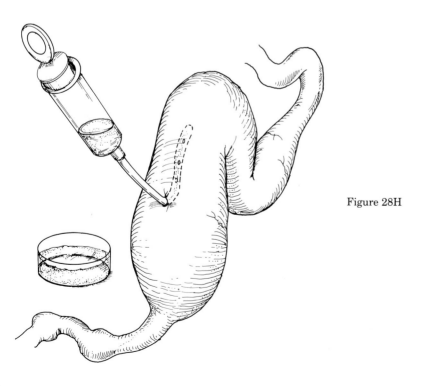

Figure 28H

Necrotizing enterocolitis

Necrotizing enterocolitis (NEC) is a disease of uncertain etiology most often seen in very small, premature infants. It may also be seen in larger infants with other surgically treated disease, notably gastroschisis, "Christmas tree" intestinal atresia, coarctation of the aorta, cyanotic congenital heart disease, or patent ductus arteriosus. Most patients with NEC do not require surgical treatment. The indications for operation are obvious perforation with free intraperitoneal air, abscess formation, and obstruction. Patients who have been successfully treated medically may go on to develop stricture formation, the treatment of which is elective resection with anastomosis. At operation, infants with active NEC are sick, septic infants often on a ventilator and often requiring maximal supportive care. The objective of the procedure should be elimination of the source of peritonitis as rapidly as possible. Because of inflammation and nutritional concerns, this most often involves exteriorization of the bowel.

The surgeon may have some idea, depending on radiographs that show a static loop of intestine or a mass, as to the location of the perforation, but in general the area can be reached by a transverse supraumbilical incision (Fig. 29A).

Irregular patches of bowel wall necrosis with pending perforation may be seen on either side of the actual perforation. The bowel wall is gray-green, and pneumatosis may be extensive (Fig. 29B). The perforation may be the size of a pin hole, or large segments of gut may have disintegrated. NEC may involve the entire large and small bowel or, much less frequently, present as an isolated perforation with normal-appearing gut elsewhere.

In favorable circumstances, an isolated perforation may be treated by resection and end-to-end anastomosis. Much more often, however, extensive resection of the necrotic gut is required. Often it is impossible to determine where the NEC process begins or ends. Under these circumstances, the safest approach is to resect the frankly necrotic gut, bringing out a proximal stoma and creating a distal mucous fistula. The proximal stoma is usually best brought out through a separate incision. A small cylinder of skin 1 cm in diameter is excised, and the fascia and peritoneum are incised. The site is best located as far away from the incision and the umbilicus and iliac crest as possible to facilitate placement of the stoma bag (Fig. 29C).

Stomas should be created with obviously viable gut, if possible. Sometimes there is so much questionably viable intestine that it is necessary to bring questionable gut out as a stoma, observing the status of its survival over the ensuing 24 to 48 hours. The intestine is brought out to extend beyond the abdominal wall about 1½ cm. The gut is sutured circumferentially to the peritoneum and posterior rectus sheath with interrupted 5-0 silk. This is frequently accomplished most easily from the inside. The stoma is then "matured" by turning back the end of the stoma, attaching the end to the skin and serosa of the most proximal bowel to form a nipple. This is done with absorbable suture (Fig. 29D).

The patient will require nutritional support, antibiotics, and general premature infant care. When intestinal function has returned and the infant's general condition permits, a barium study of the distal segment should be obtained to be sure there is not an associated stricture. If there is none, the stoma is taken down, the bowel trimmed back to good gut, and anastomosis carried out similar to that described for intestinal atresia (see Chapter 27).

The major postoperative complications center around the infant's prematurity. Ventilation is often necessary and may lead to late complications of bronchopulmonary dysplasia. Intracranial hemorrhage is sometimes seen. Recurrent NEC or extension of bowel gangrene may complicate the process of trying to establish enteral nutrition. Sepsis is common.

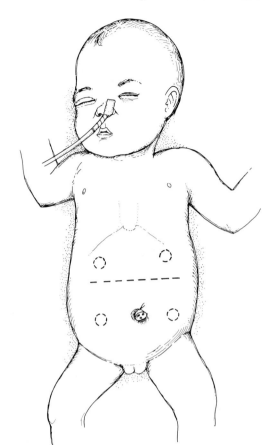

Figure 29A

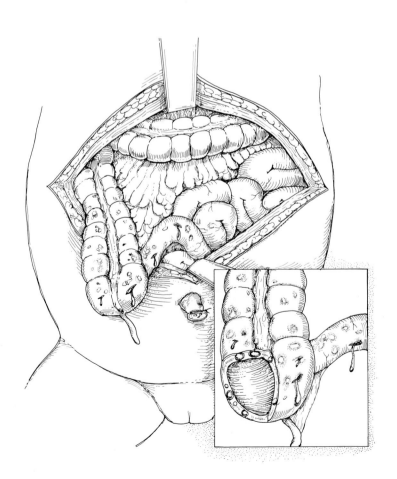

Figure 29B

Stoma takedown and restoration of gut continuity are usually elective, but a very high stoma output may necessitate early closure. Re-entry into the abdomen before 6 weeks from the time of the original procedure is usually a bloody and difficult operation. Late stoma takedown and anastomosis should be preceded by radiographic contrast study confirmation that a distal stricture is not present.

Long-term complications include adhesive obstruction and the short-gut syndrome (see Chapter 27).

Reference

Amoury RA: Necrotizing enterocolitis. In Ashcraft KW, Holder TM, eds: Pediatric Surgery. 2nd ed. Philadelphia, WB Saunders, 1993, pp 341–357.

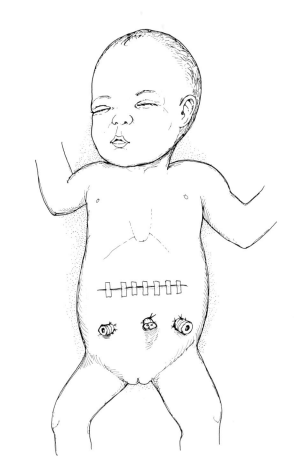

Figure 29C

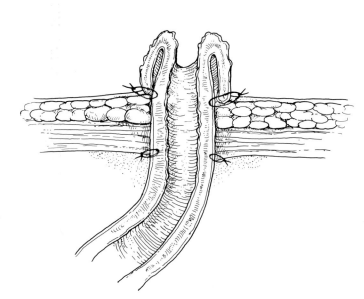

Figure 29D

Intussusception

Intussusception generally occurs when a lead point in the ileum allows peristalsis to pull the ileum into itself. Usually this progresses into the cecum. The child will have intermittent, cramping abdominal pain followed by periods of apparent complete comfort, only to have the process occur again. The most common lead point appears to be an enlarged Peyer's patch. The incidence of intussusception seems to increase during those seasons of the year when respiratory infections are more common. The typically described currant-jelly stools are usually a late phenomenon of intussusception.

Hydrostatic reduction may be accomplished in the radiology suite after the diagnosis; radiographs are used to confirm that intussusception is indeed the etiology of the patient's problem. Pneumatic reduction has been advocated by some as being less dangerous, particularly in the event of perforation of necrotic bowel. It is probably unwise to attempt either form of nonoperative reduction of the intussusception if the patient has had symptoms much longer than 48 hours or if overt bowel obstruction is present.

The operative reduction of intussusception includes preparation of the entire abdomen. A right lower quadrant transverse incision is made, much like that made for an appendectomy (Fig. 30A). The anatomy may be somewhat confusing at first, but whatever bowel presents in this region should be grasped, and usually the surgeon will see the ileum disappearing into some portion of the right colon (Fig. 30B).

The right colon should be delivered into the wound as much as possible (Fig. 30C) and the intussusception "milked" out by pushing against the intussusceptum, with very little traction placed on the ileum. Occasionally, serosal splits will occur; if this happens, frank perforation of the bowel may be impending. Great care should be taken in applying excessive pressure or tension. If the bowel is frankly necrotic, resection without reduction is safest. Spillage of intestinal content into the wound is to be avoided.

As the intussusception nears complete reduction, the tip of the appendix usually appears (Fig. 30D). It is important to ensure that the intussusception is completely reduced (Fig. 30E). The lead point, which usually will appear to be an umbilicated Peyer's patch on the terminal ileum, can often be palpated or seen. Another common lead point is Meckel's diverticulum. Uncommon lead points include polyps or tumors of the small intestine. The older the patient, the more likely the lead point is to be a tumor.

The appendix should be removed if at all possible, unless there is questionable viability of the cecum (Fig. 30F). The scar in the right lower quadrant will suggest that an appendectomy has been done, and acute appendicitis may be dismissed as impossible if the patient has a scar in this area.

The major intraoperative complication is perforation of the bowel and spillage of contents. If this occurs, the bowel should be resected back to reasonably normal bowel and an ascending ileocolostomy carried out. Sometimes it is necessary to decide whether the bowel is of such questionable viability that it ought to be resected before perforation. Usually this will occur if the intussusception symptoms have been present for more than 48 hours.

About 3% of patients who undergo an operative reduction of intussusception will have a recurrent intussusception within a few days. This is probably best managed by reoperation and resection of the lead point.

Postoperative temperature elevation to 39°C or 40°C is not unusual and is probably the result of disturbed mucosal integrity and the passage of endotoxins across the mucosal barrier. Antibiotics are probably not helpful, but in these circumstances, they cannot be avoided.

Reference

Ravitch MM: Intussusception in Infants and Children. Springfield, IL, Charles C Thomas, 1959.

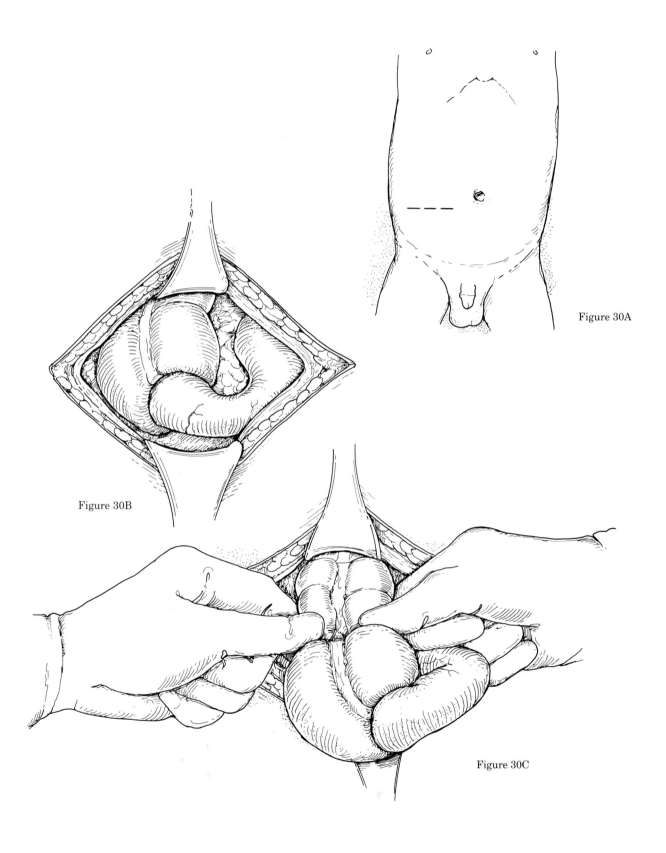

Figure 30A

Figure 30B

Figure 30C

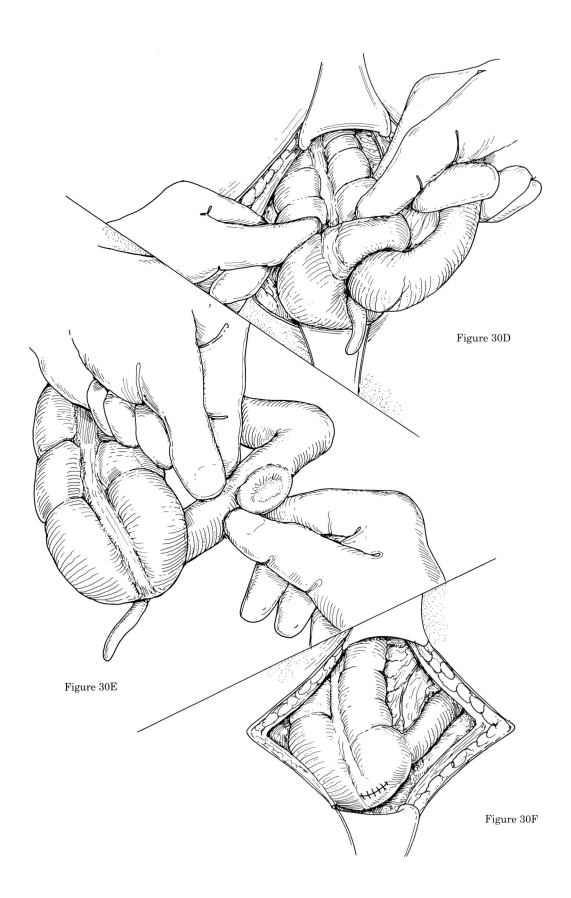

Figure 30D

Figure 30E

Figure 30F

Intestinal duplication

Intestinal duplications may occur anywhere in the gastrointestinal tract from the esophagus to the anus, but most often they occur within the abdominal cavity. Antral duplications are the most common duplications involving the stomach (Fig. 31A). They usually form a rounded mass protruding from the greater curvature of the stomach, part of which may infringe on the lumen. They usually share a common muscular wall between them, but the mucosa of the duplication is separate from the gastric mucosa of the antrum. These lesions may either be removed by resection of the mucosa from the duplication cyst, with appropriate closure of the seromuscular layer over the cavity, or by wedge resection.

Duplication cysts within the mesentery (Fig. 31B) usually produce symptoms by the accumulation of mucus in the duplication infringing on the lumen of the gut. They are best removed by wedge resection (Fig. 31C). We prefer to occlude the bowel proximally and distally with a very fine red rubber catheter passed through a mesenteric hole and snared up against a clamp. In our experience, this is the least traumatic form of bowel occlusion. The intestinal anastomosis may be carried out in a single or a double layer (see Chapter 27). The mesenteric defect should be closed to prevent herniation of the small bowel (Fig. 31D).

Sometimes there are very elongated duplications of the intestine (Fig. 31E). In these instances, complete resection of the involved normal bowel might lead to loss of more intestine than is desirable. Therefore, an alternative method of treating the duplications consists of making multiple seromuscular incisions and carefully extirpating the mucosa and submucosa from within the duplication itself (Fig. 31F).

Careful hemostasis, leaving the incisions open, will prevent development of a hematoma, which might reproduce intestinal obstruction in the postoperative period (Fig. 31G). It is probably neither necessary nor wise to try to do a long, combined anastomosis to include the duplication as part of the intestinal lumen.

Reference

Wrenn EL: Alimentary tract duplications. In Ashcraft KW, Holder TM, eds: Pediatric Surgery. 2nd ed. Philadelphia, WB Saunders, 1993, pp 421–434.

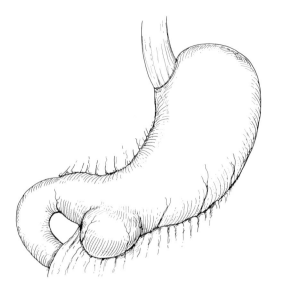

Figure 31A

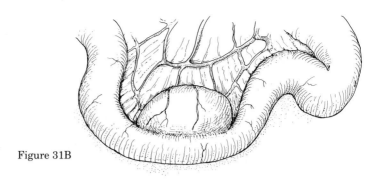

Figure 31B

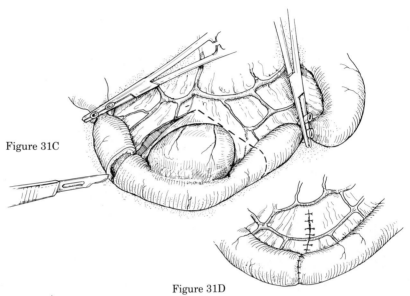

Figure 31C

Figure 31D

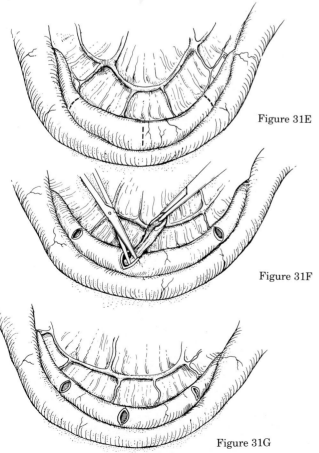

Figure 31E

Figure 31F

Figure 31G

32

Meckel's diverticulum

An outpouching in the terminal ileum known as Meckel's diverticulum exists in about 2% of the population but is asymptomatic in most people. The most common clinical presentation of Meckel's diverticulum is significant gastrointestinal bleeding, which usually occurs in childhood. The etiology of the gastrointestinal hemorrhage is peptic ulceration caused by acid production from the gastric mucosa often present in the distal end of Meckel's diverticulum. The acid creates an ulceration of the surrounding ileal mucosa. The passage of maroon blood through the rectum without the presence of blood in the stomach is strongly suggestive of Meckel's diverticulum. Inflammation of Meckel's diverticulum such as occurs in the appendix is unusual, but in most patients who undergo exploration for appendicitis and in whom a normal appendix is seen, exploration of the terminal three to four feet of ileum for the presence of a Meckel's diverticulum is warranted.

The diagnosis is usually determined by a technetium Tc 99m pertechnetate scan, as Tc 99m pertechnetate will be concentrated in gastric mucosa. False-negative and false-positive results exist, however, further confusing the clinical picture. Some of the isotope is concentrated in the urinary bladder, and very often a Meckel's diverticulum will be located very near the dome of the bladder, making differentiation difficult.

There is no question that a Meckel's diverticulum that produces bleeding should be resected, and a Meckel's diverticulum found at the time of laparotomy should be removed if there is palpable thickening of the mucosa at its tip. This usually represents ectopic gastric mucosa and a resultant likelihood of bleeding.

Meckel's diverticula most often are located on the antimesenteric border but on occasion can be on the side of the bowel or even in the mesentery itself. Meckel's diverticulum may serve as the lead point for intussusception.

Resection of a Meckel's diverticulum, which is usually a broad-based structure, should be carried out by making a longitudinally oriented enterotomy around the base of the diverticulum. We prefer to use the needlepoint electrocautery. In the case of massive gastrointestinal bleeding from the Meckel's diverticulum, the blood supply to this structure will be significant and needs ligature, if not suture ligatures, for control (Fig. 32A).

We prefer to close the longitudinal enterotomy in a transverse fashion using a continuous Connell suture placed from outside the bowel, thus closing it in one layer (Fig. 32B). In this way there will be no diminution in the diameter of the ileum.

Complications after removal of a Meckel's diverticulum are very uncommon.

Reference

Foglia RP: Meckel's diverticulum. In Ashcraft KW, Holder TM, eds: Pediatric Surgery. 2nd ed. Philadelphia, WB Saunders, 1993, pp 435–439.

Figure 32A

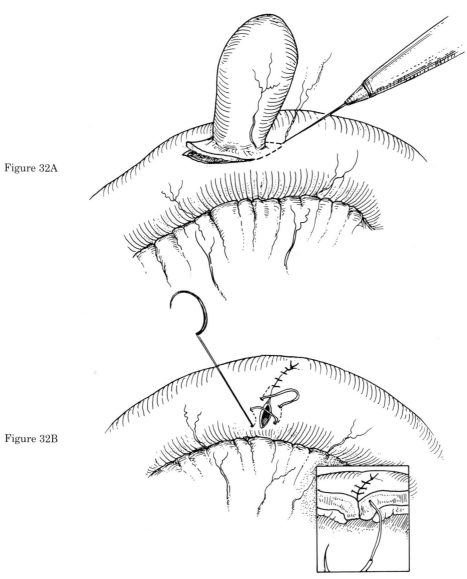

Figure 32B

CHAPTER

33

Colostomy

Temporary colostomy is most often necessary in pediatric patients to relieve obstruction caused by Hirschsprung's disease or imperforate anus. It is rarely necessary to create a permanent colostomy in children.

Several colostomy techniques are illustrated here. It is important to remember that feces delivered by the proximal stoma may pass into the distal stoma if the loop colostomy is used. If it is important that distal accumulation of stool not occur, as in the patient with imperforate anus, a loop colostomy should not be performed.

It is also important to place the stoma in such a way that an appliance may be fitted for collection of feces. For example, placement must take into account the fact that in small infants, the thighs are most often flexed onto the abdomen and in pubescent patients, pubic hair may interfere with the satisfactory application of an appliance.

LOOP COLOSTOMY

The transverse loop colostomy is performed most often in very ill infants with Hirschsprung's disease when the level of aganglionosis is not known. Because aganglionosis is limited to the sigmoid colon or rectum in the vast majority of patients with Hirschsprung's disease, it is reasonably safe to create such a colostomy when frozen section confirmation of the presence of ganglion cells is not possible.

The incision is usually a right transverse supraumbilical incision (Fig. 33A). A loop of transverse colon is exposed (Fig. 33B). The omentum is taken down from it and delivered back within the abdominal cavity. A window is then made in the mesentery, and a length of red rubber catheter is passed through. This red rubber catheter is sutured to itself to form a ring (Fig. 33C), which will prevent retraction of the loop into the abdominal cavity. Fixation at the level of the peritoneum with multiple interrupted permanent sutures is important. The gap between afferent and efferent limbs should not be too large, otherwise small bowel herniation may occur at that point.

The day after creation of this loop, the electrocautery is used to open the colon by way of a transverse incision into the lumen (Fig. 33D). Until this time the patient must be kept on nasogastric suction to prevent additional abdominal distention. The delay between operation and colostomy allows sealing of the peritoneum and is probably important in preventing peritonitis. At the time of opening the colostomy, a piece of colon may be submitted to the pathologist for pathologic confirmation of the presence of ganglion cells.

The matured stoma forms after removal of the loop of red rubber catheter on approximately the seventh day (Fig. 33E). However, stool that exudes from the working stoma may be passed into the distal stoma by natural peristaltic action.

DIVIDED COLOSTOMY

The transverse divided colostomy is probably best performed through a small vertical supraumbilical incision (Fig. 33F). The colon on either side of the middle colic vessels is brought up as a loop (Fig. 33G). Its mesentery is divided, including the arcade (Fig. 33H). Two heavy silk ligatures are tied on either side of the point where the colon is to be divided. The bowel is then divided with electrocautery. The stoma sites are prepared on either side of the midline, and each segment of colon is brought out through its respective stoma. The midline wound may then be closed (Fig. 33I). As with any stoma formation, the serosa of the bowel as it exits the abdominal wall is attached to the peritoneum with interrupted permanent sutures.

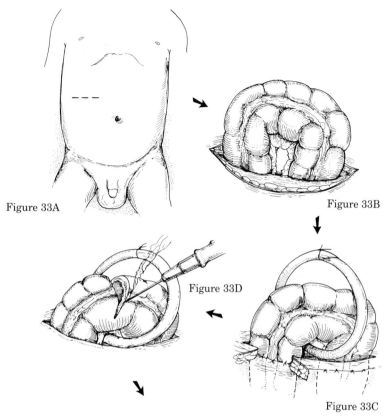

Figure 33A

Figure 33B

Figure 33D

Figure 33C

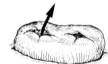

Figure 33E

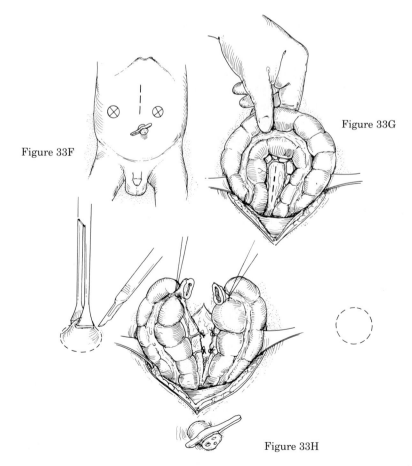

Figure 33F

Figure 33G

Figure 33H

After the midline wound is closed, the occluding ligatures are removed from the ends of the colon in turn and a mature stoma created (Fig. 33*J*). For the "maturation," we use absorbable suture, creating a nipple of sufficient length that it will fit nicely into an appliance.

LEVELING COLOSTOMY

When Hirschsprung's disease exists and colostomy is to be created at the most distal level of ganglion cells, the procedure is usually accomplished through a lower transverse abdominal incision (Fig. 33*K*). Because the majority of patients have ganglion cells in the upper sigmoid or descending colon, the stoma is usually located in the left abdomen.

Two methods of handling the distal bowel are shown. The first is an oversewn or stapled Hartmann's pouch (Fig. 33*L*), and the second is a distal mucous fistula that may be brought out through the wound, leaving a bridge of skin wide enough for the application of a bag to collect stool (Fig. 33*M*). We prefer Hartmann's pouch.

COMPLICATIONS

Complications of colostomy formation include stoma prolapse. This is usually caused by inadequate fixation of the serosa around the edges of the wound or by creating too large a fascial defect so that the more proximal colon can prolapse through the stoma. Retraction of the stoma is possible if the maturing nipple is not properly formed. Both of these complications are usually due to inadequate fixation of the serosa to the inside of the abdominal wall. The stoma is best created by excising a button of skin about 1 cm in diameter in a newborn and up to 2 cm in diameter in an older child. The fascia and muscle are then split in a cruciate manner without excision; thus the fascial defect will not be made too large.

Colostomy takedown is sometimes very difficult to perform. The dissection requires a great deal of skill to prevent the loss of more colon than is absolutely necessary. It is possible, by careful dissection, to take down a matured stoma and unfold it, allowing anastomosis of the ends of a divided colostomy with minimal resection. The needle electrocautery is most useful for this procedure.

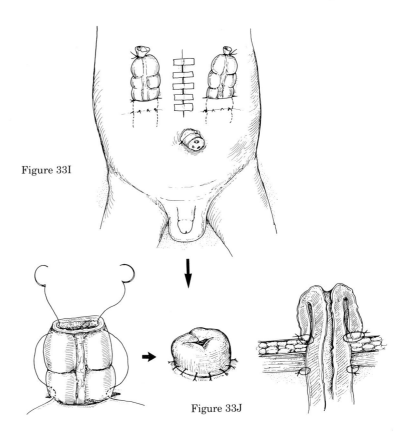

Figure 33I

Figure 33J

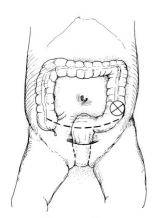

Figure 33K

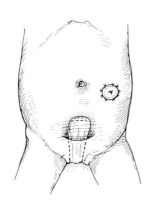

Figure 33L

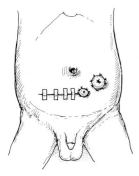

Figure 33M

Omphalocele and gastroschisis

An omphalocele is an abdominal wall defect through which the intestine and the liver may herniate into the umbilical cord (Fig. 34A), causing the cord to come off the omphalocele membrane. Very rarely, an omphalocele may rupture during the delivery process. Most are diagnosed in utero by ultrasonography, and delivery is by cesarean section.

A gastroschisis is a much smaller abdominal wall defect than an omphalocele and is located to the right of the intact umbilical cord. The majority of gastroschisis patients do not have a membrane covering the intestine (Fig. 34B). However, some have matted intestine covered by a membrane that is opaque and thick, referred to as a "peel" (Fig. 34C).

In both omphalocele and gastroschisis, the abdominal cavity is small, and the defect may not be able to be closed primarily, particularly in the case of an omphalocele. Because the abdominal wall defect is small in gastroschisis, it is often necessary to enlarge the defect by an incision upward near the midline. In approximately 50% to 70% of patients, gastroschisis can be closed primarily by enlarging the defect and then stretching the abdominal wall. This is done by placing two fingers of one hand on one side and two fingers of the other on the other side and simply stretching the wall from the inside. If the intestine can be reduced into the abdominal cavity and the defect closed without compromising ventilation owing to increased intra-abdominal pressure or producing vascular compromise by compression of the vena cava, then primary closure should be accomplished. Otherwise, a staged return of viscera to the abdominal cavity must be accomplished. As with most cases of omphalocele, a Silastic-coated, Dacron, or other synthetic mesh is used to construct a silo, suturing this to the fascia around the edges of the defect (Fig. 34D). In patients with omphalocele, the sac is left intact, thereby reducing the chance for infection. The silo is then closed up its side and across the top. An umbilical artery catheter is usually placed during the initial procedure for postoperative blood gas monitoring.

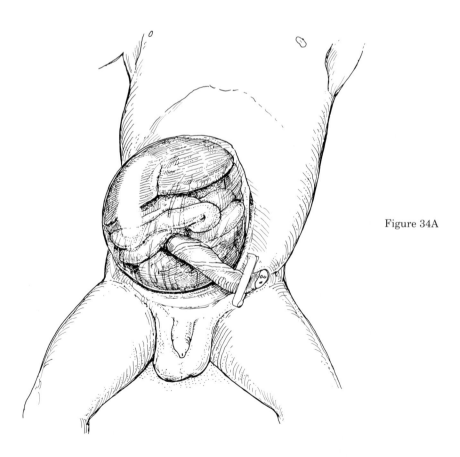

Figure 34A

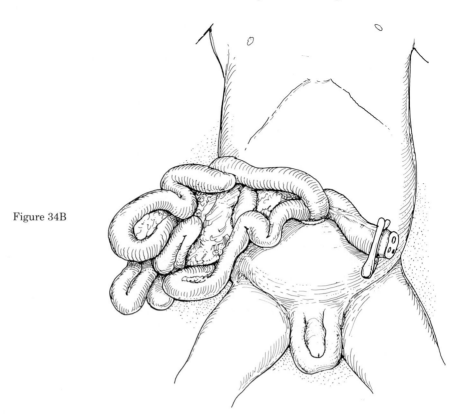

Figure 34B

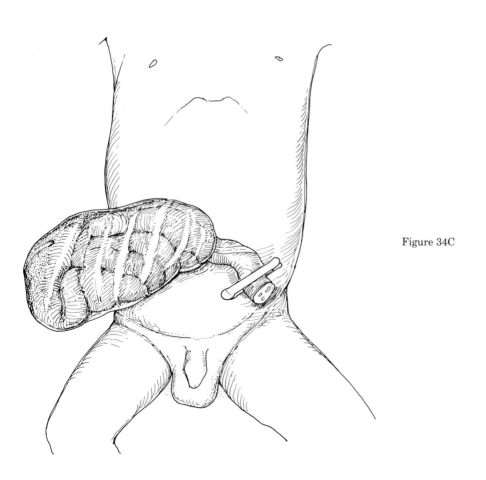

Figure 34C

Over several days, the viscera are returned to the abdominal cavity by squeezing down on the silo (Fig. 34*E*). When no more viscera can be reduced by compression of the silo, the patient is returned to the operating room to undergo removal of the silo and operative closure of the fascia. Steri-Strips are used to close the skin (Fig. 34*F*). This entire process should be accomplished in about 7 to 10 days.

In both gastroschisis and omphalocele, malrotation of the intestine is present, but it rarely is associated with duodenal bands and upper intestinal obstruction. Intestinal atresia may occur less commonly with omphalocele than with gastroschisis, but it is probably not worth opening the omphalocele membrane for exploration, as this is an uncommon phenomenon. In the patient with gastroschisis, matting and inflammation of the bowel will preclude easy delineation of bowel continuity. It is far better to reduce the abdominal contents, treat the patient with total parenteral nutrition either peripherally or centrally until bowel function returns, and then manage the intestinal continuity if problems occur.

Early postoperative complications include delayed intestinal function. If, after several weeks, the question of intestinal tract continuity is not resolved, contrast studies should be performed. We have seen surprisingly few postoperative adhesive obstructions in patients with gastroschisis or omphalocele. Although the intestine in the patient with gastroschisis seems to be foreshortened, rarely, if ever, does short-gut syndrome exist in the absence of a vascular accident or strangulation in the antenatal period.

Reference

Tunell WP: Omphalocele and gastroschisis. In Ashcraft KW, Holder TM, eds: Pediatric Surgery. 2nd ed. Philadelphia, WB Saunders, 1993, pp 546–556.

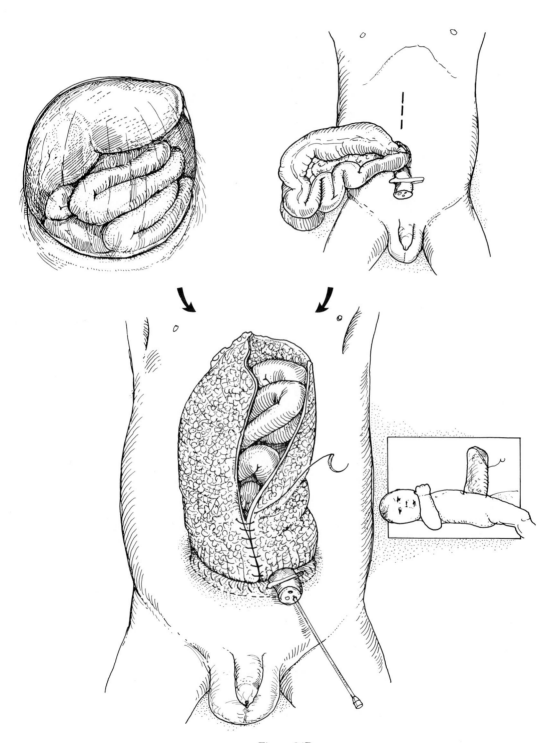

Figure 34D

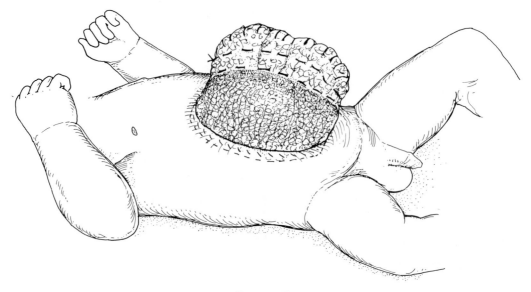

Figure 34E

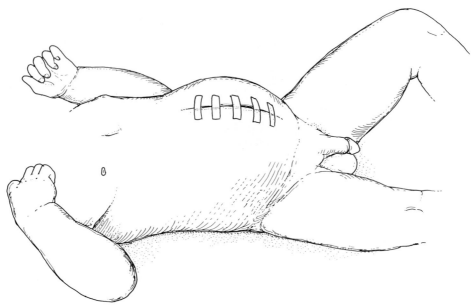

Figure 34F

35

Mini-Pena procedure

Pena procedure

Pena and de Vries devised the approach to imperforate anus that is currently the most widely practiced in pediatric surgery. This procedure is based on anatomic delineations of the musculature of continence beyond those of Stephens. The operative approach itself is based on the concept that muscles will function satisfactorily if cut and reapproximated accurately. The continence that follows repair of imperforate anus appears to be related to the patient's inherent anatomic structures, as accurate placement of the rectum within the muscle complex is currently the rule.

Figure 36A illustrates the normal anatomy in boys, showing the pelvic floor with the muscle complex extending down toward the circular external sphincter. Continence depends on the ability to elevate and anteriorly angulate the rectal canal (Fig. 36B). Because most patients with imperforate anus are born with this muscle complex intact, it is possible, with careful dissection and adequate visualization, to build a rectal canal and anus that utilize all of the potential continence mechanisms.

Boys with imperforate anus commonly have a fistula to the membranous urethra just distal to the prostate (Fig. 36C). The most common anatomic situation in girls is the rectal fourchette fistula (Fig. 36D). Less commonly seen is a fistula to the vagina above the level of the hymen (Fig. 36E).

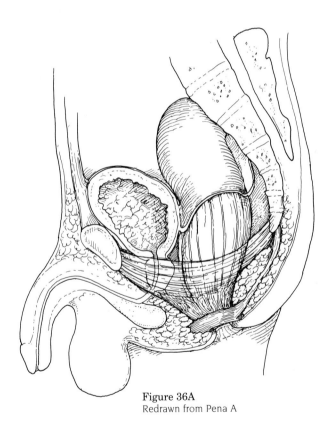

Figure 36A
Redrawn from Pena A

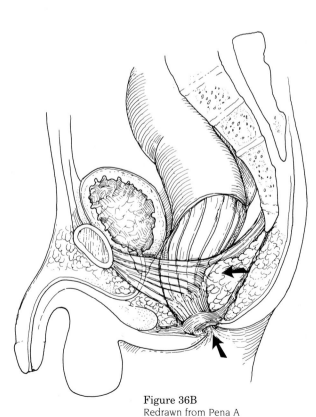

Figure 36B
Redrawn from Pena A

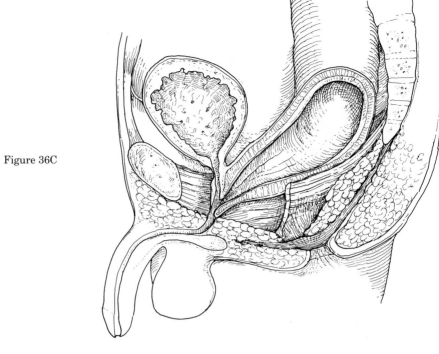

Figure 36C

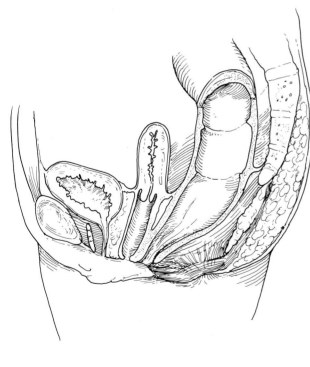

Figure 36D

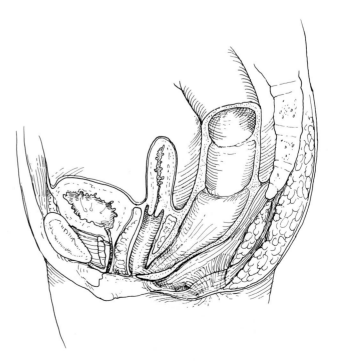

Figure 36E

In the newborn with imperforate anus, it is important to delineate the precise anatomy. This is done by inspecting and probing the perineum in girls and by performing a retrograde urethrogram in boys. The initial step in repair of the imperforate anus is to perform a divided colostomy in the newborn, most preferably in the transverse colon, so that there is a maximum amount of left colon for mobilization and repair.

The definitive procedure, commonly known as the Pena procedure, is also called a posterior sagittal anorectoplasty (PSARP). It may be performed in infants as young as 1 month of age and probably is best performed before the infant is 6 months old. The patient is positioned supine with a large, soft roll under the lower abdomen to elevate the buttocks (Fig. 36F).

A midline incision (Fig. 36G, inset) is made from the lower sacrum through the external sphincter and toward the vulva or scrotum. Electrical stimulation of the anal dimple allows precise localization of the center of the external sphincter; this should be marked before making the incision. The incision may be made with a needlepoint electrocautery or with a knife through the skin. Meticulous hemostasis aids in the delineation of the midline and in identification of the muscle complex as it is encountered. Dissection precisely in the midline reveals a thin fascia covering the pelvic fat on either side; exposed fat indicates that the dissection is not precisely on the midline. The coccyx may be split or excised, allowing access to the retrorectal space. The superficial muscle bundles that extend from the external sphincter to the deep side of the coccyx are located and, at the surgeon's discretion, may be tagged with an identifying retraction suture (Fig. 36G).

Incision of the deeper pelvic floor or levator muscle then provides access to the posterior wall of the rectum. The rectum is usually visible and palpable at this point if there is a fistulous communication to the urinary tract. In a patient without fistula, the bulbous end of the rectum may be located very high up in the wound, anterior to the sacrum. Whenever a structure suspected to be the rectum is opened, traction sutures should be placed and the opening made precisely in the midline posteriorly (Fig. 36H). In this way, closure or tapering of the rectum may be carried out directly posteriorly. Inspection of the anterior wall of the opened rectum will usually reveal a fistulous communication (Fig. 36I).

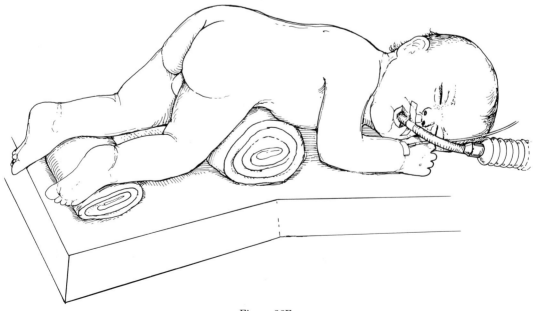

Figure 36F

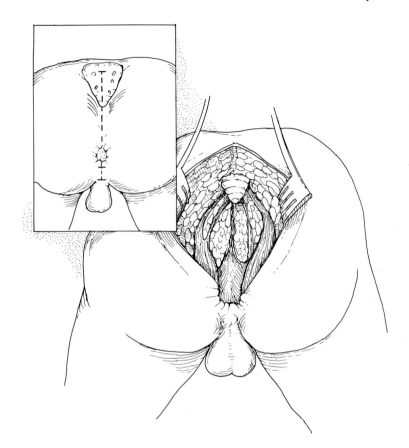

Figure 36G

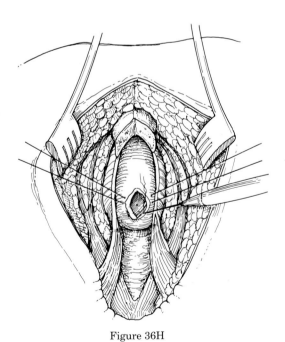

Figure 36H

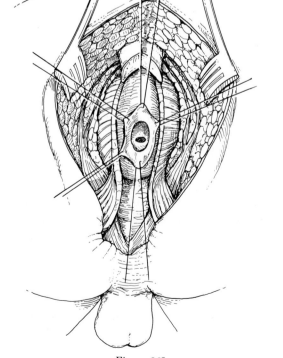

Figure 36I

Multiple traction sutures are placed around the fistula, and it is lifted and dissected from the urethra or vagina. There is no natural plane of dissection immediately cephalad to the fistula, and therefore creation of a separate rectum and vagina or urethra must be done very carefully (Fig. 36*J*, inset). The vaginal or rectourethral fistula is closed with interrupted sutures. The rectum is dissected cephalad until it is easily separable from the posterior wall of the bladder or the posterior wall of the vagina. This usually indicates that there is enough length to allow the rectum to be brought down to the site where the anus will be constructed. If there has been entry into the vagina or into the urethra during this most delicate part of the dissection, it is important that adequate closure be accomplished, again with absorbable suture. The urinary tract should be decompressed by an indwelling Foley catheter during the procedure and the immediate postoperative period.

Frequently the bulbous end of the rectum needs to be tapered to allow it to fit comfortably into the muscle complex. Tapering of the portion of the rectum that traverses the muscle complex is done by excision of a strip of rectum posteriorly (Fig. 36*K*). The reduced rectum is then closed with posterior interrupted permanent sutures so that it can be trimmed to length without disrupting a continuous suture line (Fig. 36*L*). The muscle complex is closed anteriorly to separate the rectum from the urinary tract.

The tapered rectum is laid into the muscle complex, and the muscle complex, including the levators and the external sphincter, is closed posteriorly (Fig. 36*M*). Tapering of the rectum allows closure of the muscle complex without excessive tension. We prefer to excise two small diamonds of skin, as described by Nixon, and to shorten the pulled-through rectum so that as the neoanus is created, the two side flaps of skin are pulled up into the perineum (Fig. 36*N*).

The neoanus is constructed with permanent Prolene suture. The lateral points of the diamonds are brought together to aid in creating an anus that exposes no mucosa. Subcuticular closure of the posterior midline skin incision follows the closure of the superficial muscle complex. The patient is discharged the day of operation or the following day and returns for removal of the anal sutures under general anesthesia 2 weeks later, at which time the first rectal dilatation is accomplished.

We prefer the first dilatation to be done with a No. 8 Hegar. Parents are instructed to repeat this dilatation daily for 1 week, at which time they turn the Hegar to the No. 9 end and dilate for a week. They then return to ensure that the dilatations are being carried out satisfactorily and are then given a No. 10 and No. 11 Hegar. After 2 weeks of progressive daily dilatations, the No. 12 Hegar is used. Plans are then made for colostomy closure.

Complications of this or any other anoplasty include mucocutaneous stricture and mucosal prolapse. Regular dilatation is most likely to prevent the former, and the latter is made less likely by Nixon's modification in the anoplasty.

After closure of the colostomy, excoriation of the perianal skin is often seen. This may be ameliorated by application of cholestyramine ointment (15% in a cholesterolized anhydrous petrolatum [Aquaphor] base) or by the use of milk of magnesia applied topically to the area after each stool. This is usually a self-limiting disorder but can be very distressing for both parents and children.

Long-term function after the PSARP appears to be as good or better than any anoplastic technique previously described. However, patients with an abnormal sacrum are less likely to have good control. In patients with serious sacral deformities, consideration should be given to permanent colostomy without any attempt to build an anus. Few things are worse than an uncontrollable perineal colostomy.

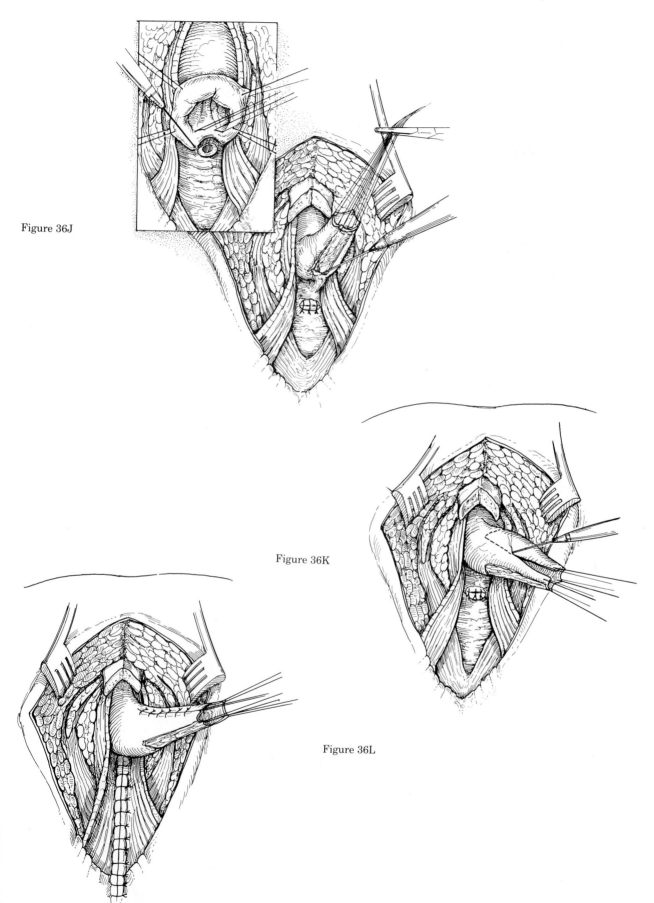

Figure 36J

Figure 36K

Figure 36L

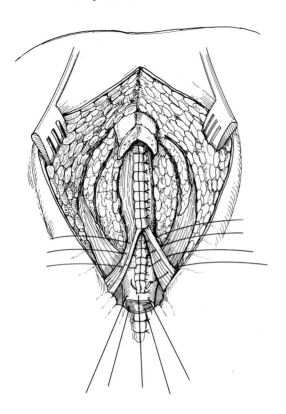

Figure 36M

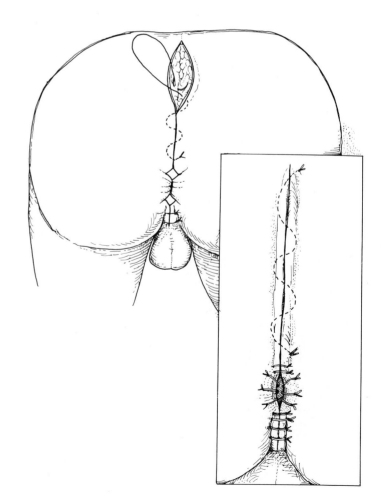

Figure 36N

References

de Vries P, Pena A: Posterior sagittal anorectoplasty. J Pediatr Surg 17:638–643, 1982.

Nixon HH: Imperforate anus. British surgical practice. In Surgical Progress. Butterworth & Co, London, 1961.

Pena A: Atlas of Surgical Management of Anorectal Malformations. Springer-Verlag, New York, 1990.

Pena A, de Vries P: Posterior sagittal anorectoplasty. Important technical considerations and new applications. J Pediatr Surg 17:796–881, 1982.

Stephens FD: Imperforate rectum: A new surgical technique. Med J Aust 1:202–206, 1953.

Soave pull-through

A pull-through operative procedure for the correction of Hirschsprung's disease requires access from both the abdominal cavity and the anus. We prefer to prepare the patient sterilely from the nipple line down to the mid thigh. The feet, legs, and thighs are then wrapped with sterile dressings so that they may be laid onto the sterile field and moved up and down as needed. This technique of draping, referred to as the "Chinese technique," allows the patient to be lifted up or laid down completely supine. It also allows the patient to be positioned so that access to the abdomen or the anus is easily managed by the surgeons, and one can go back and forth without difficulty (Figs. 37A, 37B).

If the patient has already undergone a leveling colostomy and creation of a Hartmann's pouch, attention is turned to the pelvis. A lower abdominal transverse incision is used. The outer longitudinal and inner circular muscles of the rectal stump are incised, taking care to remain in the submucosal plane outside the lumen for the dissection. If the bowel is intact, this incision is made at about the level of the peritoneal reflection or a little lower (Fig. 37C). Scissors or a blunt dissector may be used to develop the plane. The presence of ganglion cells must be determined in these patients in order to select the bowel for pull-through.

Some surgeons prefer to inject saline or saline mixed with diluted epinephrine solution to enhance the dissection by hydrodissection and to reduce capillary bleeding. This dissection should be carried down as far as possible. Stretching of the aganglionic rectal muscle sleeve during this dissection helps to reduce its obstructive potential postoperatively.

Once the dissection has proceeded as far into the pelvis as possible (which can be determined by inserting one palpating finger into the dissection and one into the anus), the dissection is started from below (Fig. 37D). An incision about 1 cm above the dentate line is made circumferentially around the rectum, and blunt and sharp dissection are used to complete the endorectal dissection. Care must be taken to remove all the mucosa and not to leave patches; otherwise, a mucocele will develop between the serosa of the pulled-through colon and the aganglionic muscular sleeve of the rectum. We prefer to split the aganglionic rectal sleeve posteriorly to reduce the obstructive capabilities of this aganglionic segment (Fig. 37E). We then pull through the normal ganglionated bowel and suture the full thickness of the ganglionated bowel to the mucosal edge above the dentate line. Placement of these sutures is facilitated by placing traction sutures laterally at the mucocutaneous junction; these are then passed through the buttock skin and tied sufficiently tight to somewhat evert the anus. Accurately placed quadrant sutures provide an additional source of traction, enhancing exposure. Several interrupted sutures are used to fix the pulled-through bowel to the upper edge of the aganglionic muscle sleeve. The muscle sleeve should probably be made as short as possible to obviate obstructing the bowel.

Soave's original description did not include the distal anastomosis. The pulled-through, ganglionated bowel was allowed to protrude through the anus and form an adhesive union to the muscle cuff. Ten to 14 days later, the patient underwent trimming of this segment and anastomosis to the rectal mucosa. A primary distal anastomosis, proposed by Boley, eliminates the discomfort and the very foul smelling serositis of the exposed aganglionated bowel.

The primary complication of the Soave procedure is obstruction, which may lead to obstipation and even to severe enterocolitis.

A cuff abscess or a mucocele that develops between the cuff and the pull-through is usually a result of leaving a small patch of mucosa. This may be exceedingly troublesome. Because the Soave procedure is technically more demanding and takes much longer to perform, the Duhamel procedure (see Chapter 38) seems to be preferred by the majority of pediatric surgeons at present.

References

Boley SJ: New modification of the surgical treatment of Hirschsprung's disease. Surgery 56:1015, 1964.

Duhamel B: Retrorectal and transanal pull-through procedure for the treatment of Hirschsprung's disease. Dis Colon Rectum 7:455, 1964.

Soave F: A new surgical technique for treatment of Hirschsprung's disease. Surgery 56:1007, 1964.

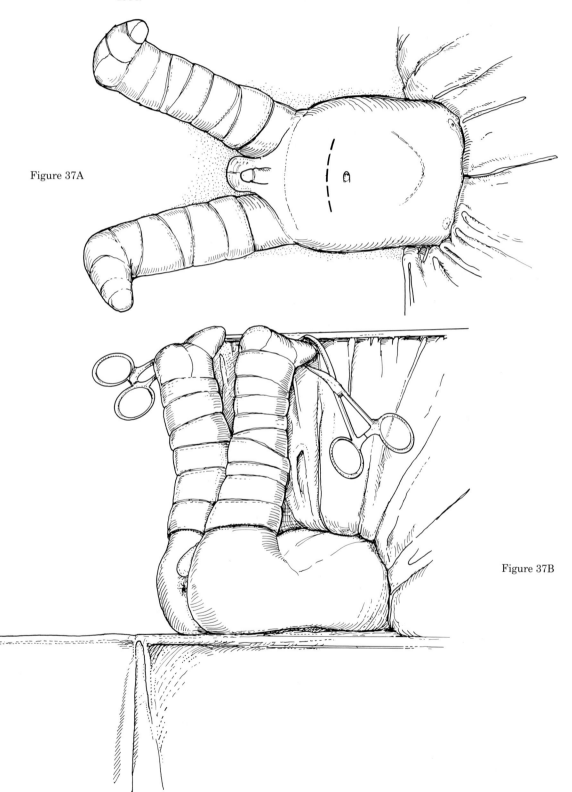

Figure 37A

Figure 37B

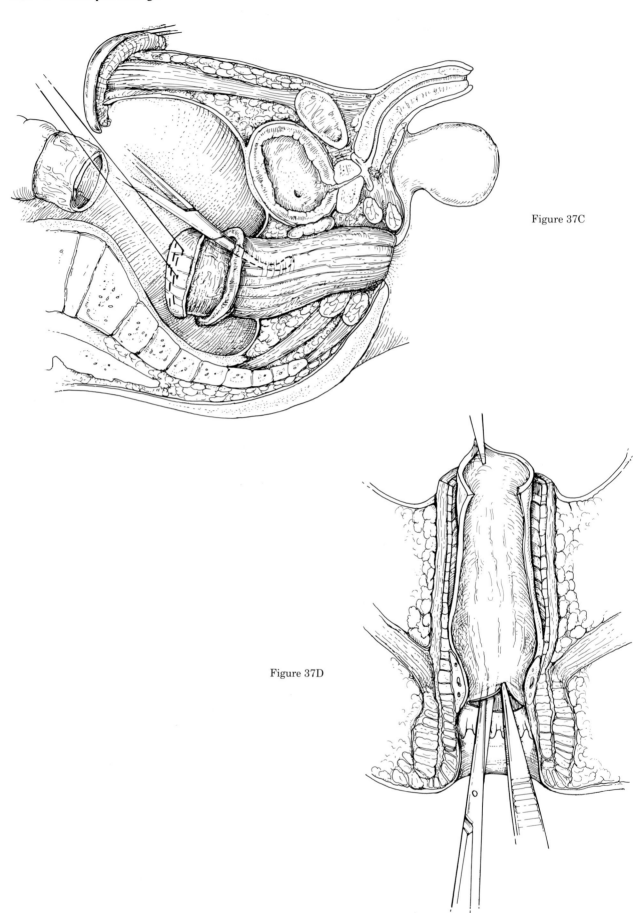

Figure 37C

Figure 37D

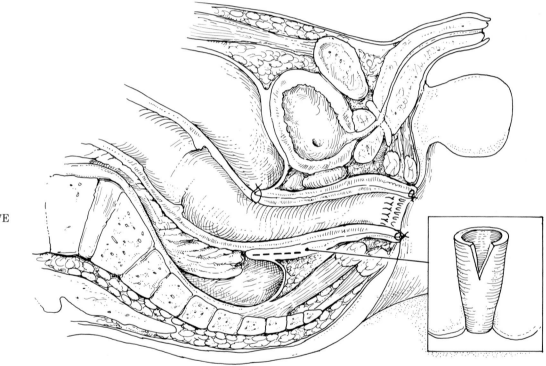

Figure 37E

38

Duhamel procedure

The Duhamel procedure is probably the most commonly performed procedure for Hirschsprung's disease worldwide because of its technical ease.

If the patient has already undergone a leveling colostomy and creation of a Hartmann's pouch, the procedure will not require pathologic determination of the presence or absence of ganglion cells. If the patient has an intact colon, then frozen section determination of the distal level of ganglion cells must be done. There must be no mistake about having ganglionated bowel for the anastomosis, because a repeat operation is impossible.

The patient is positioned supine and prepped and draped in the "Chinese" fashion shown for the Soave procedure (see Chapter 37). A transverse incision is made in the abdomen below the umbilicus. For the perineal portion, the legs are raised and fastened temporarily to an ether screen (Figs. 38A, 38B).

On entering the abdomen, the colostomy stoma is detached from the abdominal wall with the needle electrocautery and the abdominal wall defect closed in anatomic layers. The stoma is closed with several sutures and the ends left long for subsequent use to pull the colon through to the perineum. The colon is mobilized so that the stoma will reach the perineum without tension and with an unimpaired blood supply.

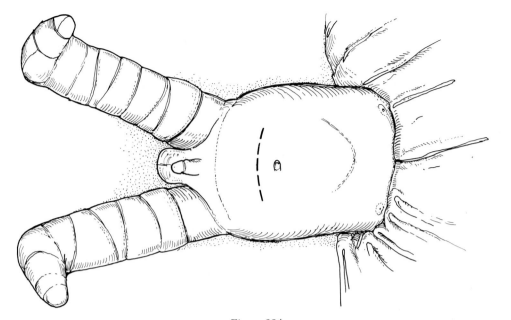

Figure 38*A*

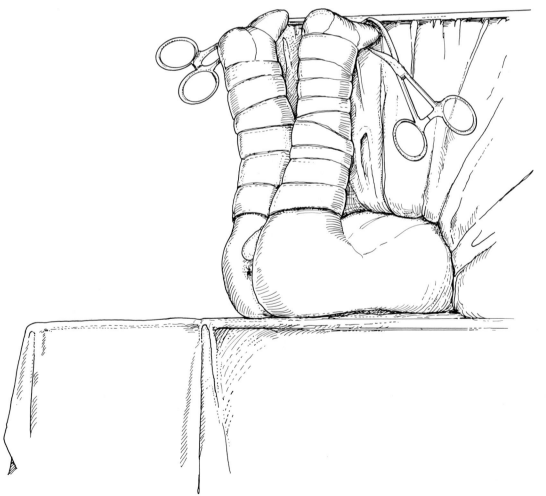

Figure 38*B*

In the Duhamel procedure, a long Hartmann's pouch is not of much concern, because the upper portion of it will be trimmed after the staple anastomosis. However, a pouch that is too short makes the pelvic procedure more difficult. Traction sutures should be placed on the Hartmann's pouch and sharp dissection used to enter the rectorectal space. Blunt dissection by spreading or with a peanut dissector is then carried down to the level of the sphincters, or about ½ cm above the dentate line (Fig. 38C).

With the dissector or an assistant's finger as far down in the pelvis as possible, the legs are elevated and a transverse incision made across the posterior wall of the aganglionic rectum just above the dentate line and through the full thickness of the rectal wall, connecting with the rectorectal dissection from above (Fig. 38D). Lateral traction sutures as described in the Soave procedure (see Chapter 37) are also helpful in exposure in this procedure. Full-thickness traction sutures are placed at the lateral corner of this incision. The surgeon passes a Péan clamp through the rectal incision while an assistant loads the proximal bowel traction suture into the clamp. The ganglionic bowel is then delivered through this transverse incision (Fig. 38E). The assistant ensures that the mesocolon on the ganglionated bowel is posteriorly oriented so that the blood supply to the pulled-through segment will not be violated by stapling. Care must also be taken to avoid a 360-degree twist of the bowel.

Discarding the colostomy portion, an incision is made transversely across the posterior half of the ganglionated colon (Fig. 38F), with interrupted absorbable sutures placed at the lateral extremities of this incision. Traction allows the remaining sutures to be placed between the interrupted sutures to complete the posterior half of the anastomosis (Fig. 38G). The remaining

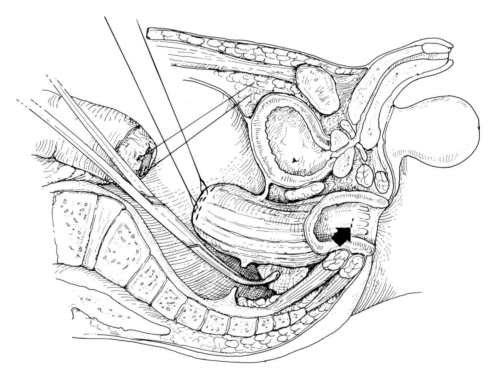

Figure 38C

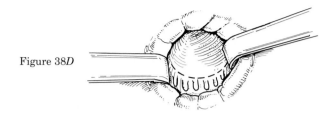

Figure 38*D*

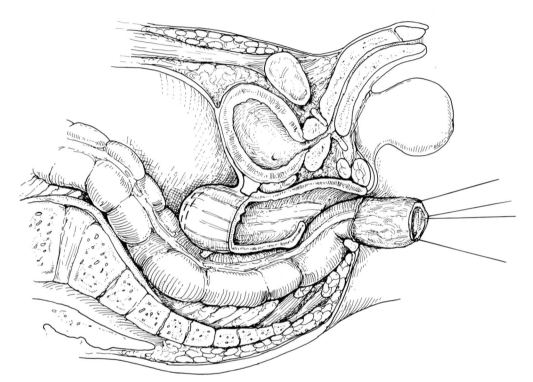

Figure 38*E*

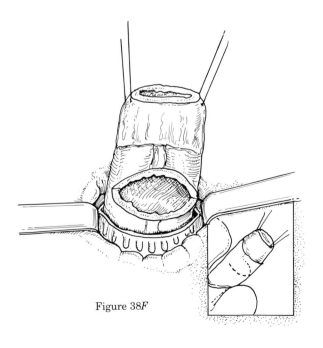

Figure 38*F*

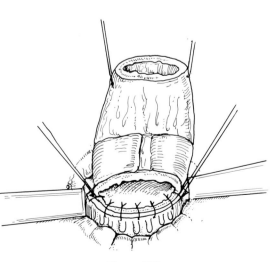

Figure 38*G*

portion of the ganglionated colon is then trimmed anteriorly. Interrupted sutures are placed to complete the circumferential anastomosis (Fig. 38*H*). The two sutures closest to the midline anteriorly are left long for retraction. The 8.5-cm or 10-cm GIA stapler is inserted directly up the Hartmann's pouch and the ganglionated colon (Fig. 38*I*). During this maneuver, the assistant again ensures that there is no twist in the colon as it comes into the pelvis and that nothing has gotten between the ganglionated colon and the aganglionic Hartmann's pouch.

The stapler is then used to anastomose the posterior ganglionated bowel with the anterior aganglionated Hartmann's pouch (Fig. 38*J*). One staple application is all that is possible from below. Use of the 8.5-cm stapler gives an adequate anastomosis up to the level of the peritoneal reflection or slightly above. In the patient with total colon aganglionosis in whom the small intestine is to be pulled through, some surgeons prefer to apply the stapler once or twice from above, leaving a much longer aganglionated rectosigmoid for absorptive purposes; this is known as the Martin procedure. Extended follow-up of patients with total colon aganglionosis has shown that one application of the stapler from below is probably all that is necessary.

The completed lower part of the anastomosis is shown from below in Figure 38*K*.

The patient's legs are then laid out flat, and the lower abdomen is approached again. The upper end of the Hartmann's pouch is trimmed obliquely

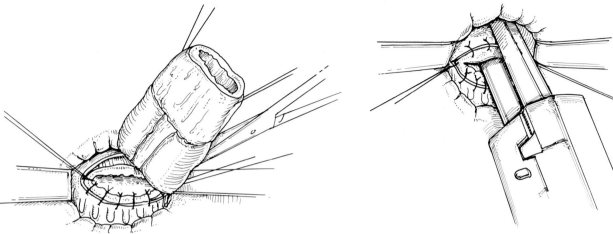

Figure 38H

Figure 38I

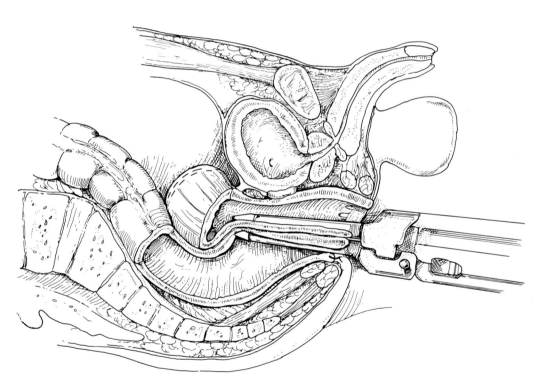

Figure 38J

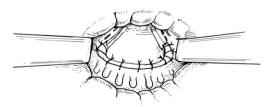

Figure 38K

down to where the staple line has ascended into the pelvis (Fig. 38*L*). Lateral corner stitches are positioned to prevent traction on the staple line. The end of the rectal pouch is then sutured to the side of the posterior ganglionic colon, completing the side-to-side anastomosis with interrupted sutures (Fig. 38*M*). These may be either permanent or absorbable. It is important not to leave any redundancy of the aganglionic rectal pouch, or a "fecaloma" may develop.

The technical pitfalls with the Duhamel procedure involve adequate posterior dissection. This dissection must extend farther down into the pelvis than one might first imagine. The second pitfall is improper alignment of the pulled-through colon. If the mesenteric border is placed in opposition to the aganglionic rectum for the staple anastomosis, the blood supply may be seriously compromised. Care must be taken not to have a 360-degree twist in the bowel before its being pulled through. Once the stapler is used to create the anastomosis, it is impossible to take the anastomosis down and redo it with sutures.

The Chinese cannot afford staplers and instead have crushed out this common wall with a specially designed ring clamp. This creates an adequate anastomosis, but it does require the patient to live with the crushing clamp up the anus for 10 to 14 days. This procedure also requires a protective colostomy or ileostomy to divert the fecal stream or an extended period of total parenteral nutrition.

Intermediate complications include bleeding from granulation tissue along the staple anastomosis. Usually this is not a significant problem. Rectal examination ought to be done before the patient's discharge from the hospital to ensure that the raw edges of the stapled anastomosis have not formed adhesions of one side to the other. Rectal dilatation also may be necessary for the first several weeks to prevent this occurrence.

Development of a fecaloma in the upper aganglionic rectal pouch has virtually disappeared as a complication since the upper end of the rectal pouch has been included in the anastomosis. The usual sort of perianal excoriation that follows takedown of a colostomy occurs with these patients. This is especially true when a great deal of the colon has been removed and its absorptive capacity reduced.

Some surgeons have recommended the use of a right colon patch on the pulled-through small intestine in total colon aganglionosis as a solution to the problem of too-liquid stools and unabsorbed bile salts. This increases the complexity of the procedure but may be worthwhile.

References

Duhamel B: Retrorectal and transanal pull-through procedure for the treatment of Hirschsprung's disease. Dis Colon Rectum 7:455, 1964.

Swenson O, Raffensperger JG: Hirschsprung's disease. In Raffensperger JG, ed: Swenson's Pediatric Surgery. 5th ed. East Norwalk, CT, Appleton & Lange, 1990, pp 556–577.

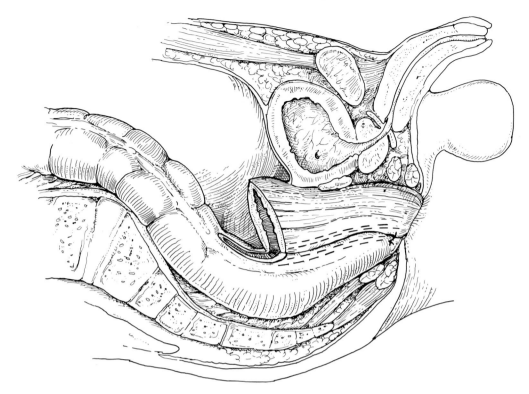

Figure 38*L*

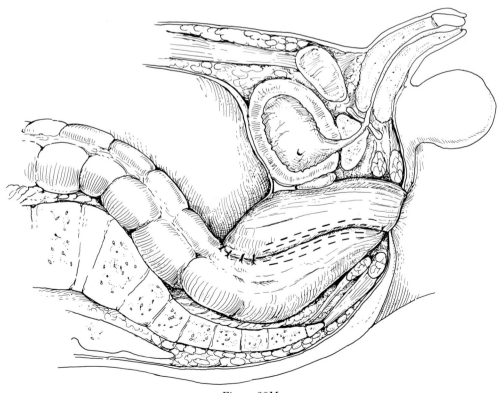

Figure 38*M*

Rectal prolapse

Prolapse of the rectum through the anus may be associated with either constipation or diarrhea. It is often seen with cystic fibrosis. A common feature in nearly all of these patients is that they spend an inordinate amount of time on the toilet. Constant straining probably stretches the rectal suspension mechanism and produces prolapse.

Intussusception of the sigmoid colon may be confused with rectal prolapse. Palpation of a short sulcus alongside the prolapse confirms that the problem is indeed rectal prolapse.

The cutaway drawing in Figure 39A depicts the rectum prolapsing or herniating through the levator sling and sphincter. With a true rectal prolapse, the examining finger alongside the prolapse can be inserted to about the dentate line.

The operation is done with the patient prone over a roll. Incision is made from the mid sacrum down to below the tip of the coccyx, staying well away from the anus (Fig. 39B). A 10-mm Hegar dilator or a No. 30 French Robinson catheter inserted to the rectum via the anus and taped in place aids in palpation of the rectum. The coccyx is removed, and the retrorectal space superior to the levators is entered (Fig. 39C). The enlarged hiatus in the levator musculature through which the rectum passes is freed, the rectum retracted anteriorly, and the levator approximated posteriorly with a series of interrupted nonabsorbable sutures (Fig. 39D). The rectum is then sutured to the levator mechanism through its posterior half with a series of interrupted sutures. The rectum is then pulled taut superiorly and sutured to the presacral fascia with several nonabsorbable sutures. The wound is then closed.

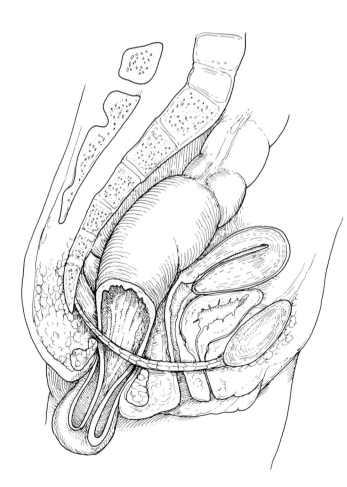

Figure 39A
Redrawn from Ashcraft KW, Amoury RA, Holder TM: Levator repair and posterior suspension for rectal prolapse. J Pediatr Surg 12:241–245, 1977.

The completed levator repair and rectal suspension are shown in Figure 39E with a portion of the rectum deleted to show the placement of the sutures.

The most likely complication is recurrence of the prolapse. In approximately 10% of our patients the prolapse recurrence proved to be a sigmoid intussusception, which was treated by sigmoid resection. Patients with caudal agenesis and a "flat bottom" are unlikely to be helped by this operation.

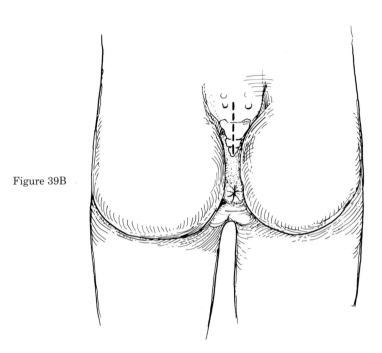

Figure 39B

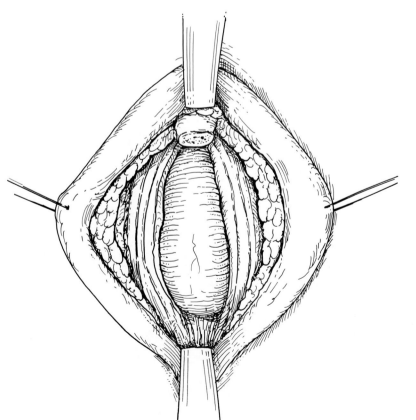

Figure 39C

References

Ashcraft KW, Holder TM: Acquired anorectal disorders. In Ashcraft KW, Holder TM, eds: Pediatric Surgery. 2nd ed. Philadelphia, WB Saunders, 1993, pp 410–415.

Ashcraft KW, Garred JL, Holder TM: Rectal prolapse—17 year experience with the posterior repair and suspension. J Pediatr Surg 25:992–995, 1990.

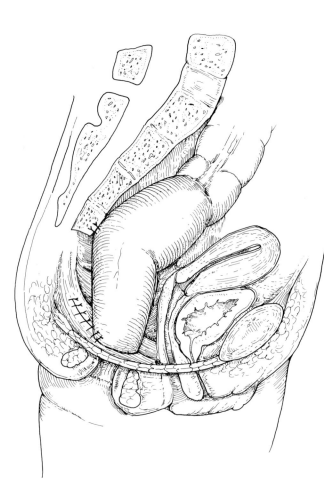

Figure 39D
Redrawn from Ashcraft KW, Amoury RA, Holder TM: Levator repair and posterior suspension for rectal prolapse. J Pediatr Surg 12:241–245, 1977.

Figure 39E
Redrawn from Ashcraft KW, Amoury RA, Holder TM: Levator repair and posterior suspension for rectal prolapse. J Pediatr Surg 12:241–245, 1977.

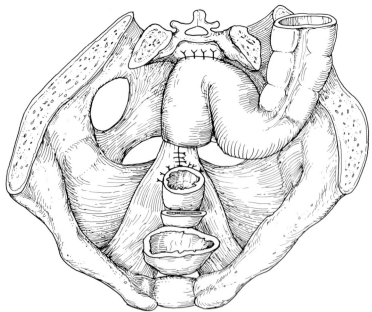

40

Sacrococcygeal teratoma

Sacrococcygeal teratomas vary in size from those that are not noted at birth to ones that are larger than the residual infant. These lesions have a malignant potential, and it is essential to remove the coccyx, because it may be the site of residual teratoma. Solid tumors are more likely to be malignant than those that are purely cystic. Although a very small teratoma may be removed with a vertical midline incision, the majority are best approached through a chevron incision.

The patient is placed supine with the thighs slightly flexed by a roll placed under the lower abdomen. In patients with very large tumors, it is helpful to pack the rectum with petrolatum gauze to help in its identification in the depths of the operative field at the time of resection. These tumors are often quite vascular.

A chevron incision is made, keeping in mind the amount of skin that must be preserved for wound closure at the termination of the procedure. Usually the point of the chevron is at the midpoint of the sacrum (Fig. 40A).

The incision is carried through the skin, subcutaneous tissue, and muscle cephalad to the tumor. Large surface vessels require careful hemostasis (Fig. 40B).

When the sacrum is reached, the entire coccyx is removed with the specimen. In the older child, transection may require an osteotome, but in most infants the coccyx may be transected with scissors or an electrocautery (Fig. 40C).

Just deep to the sacrum is the middle sacral artery, which should be identified and ligated before division. This is the primary blood supply to the teratoma.

Any presacral extension is identified and resected with the specimen (Fig. 40D). Care should be taken to avoid entering the vagina or rectum. These structures may be displaced far from their normal positions, so absolute identification is important.

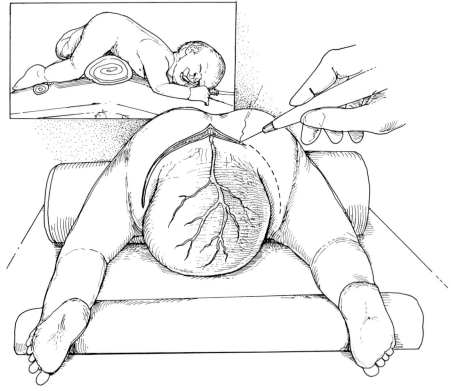

Figure 40A

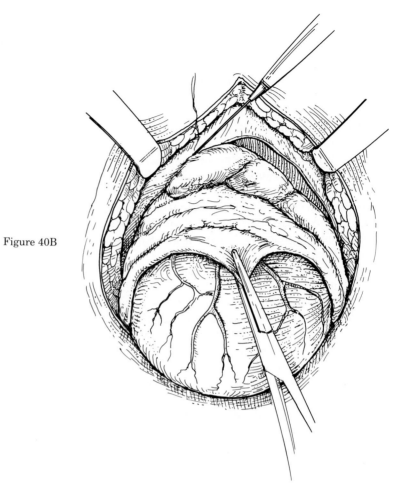

Figure 40B

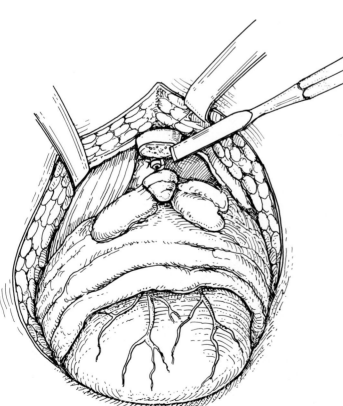

Figure 40C

The distinction between tumor and normal muscle tissue is usually not difficult. Dissection should be close to the tumor to preserve as much functioning pelvic muscle as feasible. On occasion, presacral and abdominal extension is such that a combined abdominal and sacral approach is necessary. If, on rectal examination, a palpating finger extends above the tumor, then the tumor is usually resectable by the sacral approach only. If it can be determined preoperatively that a combined approach is necessary, it is best to carry out the abdominal portion first, ligating the middle sacral vessels. The abdominal wound is closed and the patient positioned as previously indicated.

The tumor is then removed en bloc, preserving sufficient skin inferiorly to approximate the superior portion of the chevron incision. The levator muscles are approximated in the midline posteriorly and the gluteal muscles approximated in as nearly a normal position as possible. The subcutaneous tissue and skin are then closed leaving a drain in place (Fig. 40E). The baby is nursed on its abdomen for the first few days. Levator, sphincter, and gluteal muscle activity is usually satisfactory.

On occasion, transection of the coccyx will disclose an amorphous extension of tumor into the sacrum. This tissue should be removed as much as possible with a curette and submitted separately for pathologic examination. Radical removal of the sacrum is not justified at this time.

Histologic determination of malignancy may be difficult. Immature tissues, which are sometimes malignant, produce alpha-fetoprotein (AFP). Serum AFP levels should be obtained before operation and again afterward at monthly or bimonthly intervals. A very marked increase in AFP concentration is common even in benign sacrococcygeal teratomas, but a return to normal levels suggests that all the teratoma has been removed. Subsequent elevation usually means a malignant recurrence.

The major complications of sacrococcygeal teratoma resection are disturbances of bladder and bowel innervation. Preoperative studies are of no value in predicting the outcome of surgical extirpation.

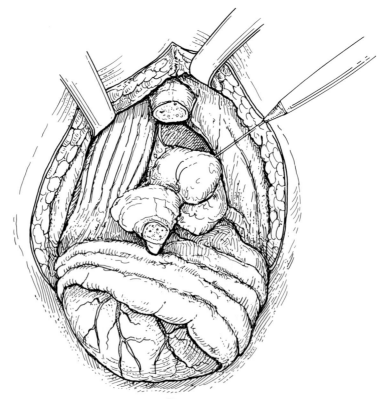

Figure 40D

Reference

Woolley MM: Teratomas. In Ashcraft KW, Holder TM, eds: Pediatric Surgery. 2nd ed. Philadelphia, WB Saunders, 1993, pp 847–862.

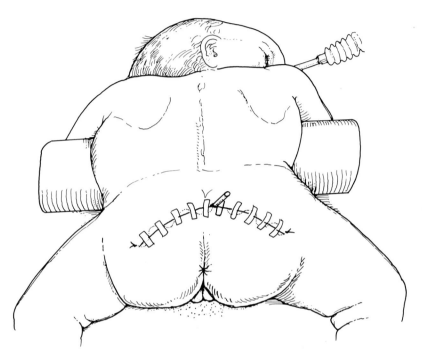

Figure 40E

Presacral teratoma

There is a variety of teratoma located in the presacral space that may occur sporadically or in a definite familial pattern. The tumors apparently are inherited as an autosomal dominant trait. They are universally associated with a defect in the sacrum (Fig. 41A) and may be intimately attached to the dura, to the posterior rectal wall, or to both. Newborns with this lesion very often have a very tight anal stenosis. Many present with intractable constipation or with an abscess in the retrorectal area involving the teratoma. Discovery of the teratoma is delayed because of the inability to insert a finger into the rectum. In the patient suspected of having a presacral teratoma and in whom anal stenosis prevents adequate examination, a "bimanual" palpation can be accomplished using a hemostat gently inserted into the anus with two palpating fingers overlying the sacrum and coccyx (Fig. 41B). With the present availability of computed tomographic (CT) scanning and magnetic resonance imaging (MRI), this diagnostic maneuver is not as important as formerly, but the impression of a mass within the hollow of the sacrum can still be gained.

The tumor is removed through a midline incision posterior to the anus. The coccyx should certainly be removed with the tumor; it may also be necessary to resect part of the posterior rectal wall to ensure that all of the tumor is removed (Fig. 41C). In such instances, after closing the rectum posteriorly, it is advisable to turn the patient over and perform a diverting colostomy. If a CT or MRI scan shows that the tumor is an integral part of the rectal wall, it may be wise to perform a diverting colostomy before the surgical approach to the teratoma. The distal bowel may then be cleansed before excision of the teratoma. Connections to the dura are closed in a watertight fashion.

It is important that all family members be examined both rectally and radiographically to determine whether the sacral defect is present and a teratoma can be palpated. A rectal examination is normally performed with the palpating portion of the index finger pointed anteriorly rather than posteriorly. These tumors will not be palpated unless the finger is turned toward the coccyx. Teratomas often appear as small discoid lesions perhaps 2 to 3 cm in diameter by 1.5 cm in thickness. Unless the patient is too old or infirm to undergo resection of an incidentally found tumor, the tumor should be removed. A parent of one of our initial patients died at age 30 as a result of malignant change in her teratoma.

The potential complications of this kind of teratoma and its resection are disturbance in the integrity of the posterior rectal wall and perhaps interference with the pelvic nerves to the bladder. All but one of these lesions have proved to be benign, and therefore a wide resection as if the lesion were malignant is not indicated.

Reference

Ashcraft KW, Holder TM, Harris DJ: Familial presacral teratomas. In New Chromosomal and Malformation Syndromes. Birth Defects Original Article Series, Vol XI. The National Foundation of the March of Dimes. 1975, pp 143–146.

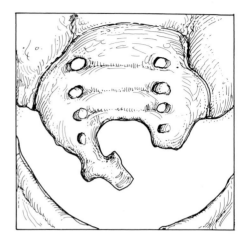

Figure 41A

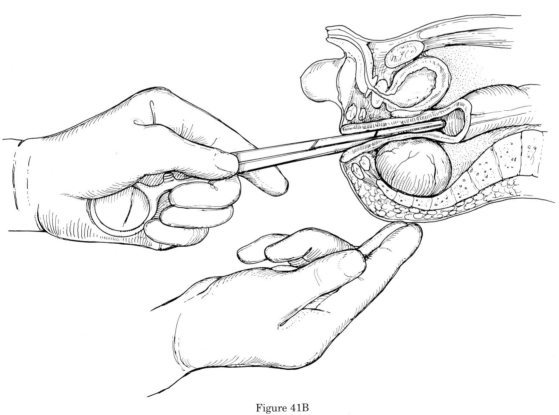

Figure 41B

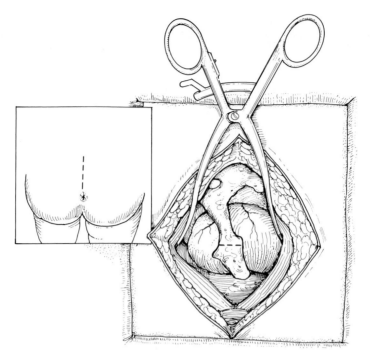

Figure 41C

42

Fistula-in-ano

Fistula-in-ano is the end result of a crypt abscess that fails to heal after spontaneous or surgical drainage. They occur most commonly in males, and it is postulated that they arise because the crypts of Morgagni are inherently abnormal.

A perirectal abscess that recurs after drainage is probably an indication that a tract lined with granulation tissue exists and that further attempts at conservative or nonsurgical therapy will be futile. In our experience, approximately 50% of perirectal abscesses continue on to fistula-in-ano. There is a small punctate lesion, usually lateral to the anus on either side (Fig. 42A). The cross-sectional view will indicate a tunnel extending through part of the anal sphincter to the dentate line (Fig. 42A, inset).

The surgical treatment of fistula-in-ano consists of placing the patient in the lithotomy or jackknife position. With the patient under general anesthesia, a probe is passed, and the orifice of the fistula is dissected sharply. The tissue lying superficial to the fistula is incised, and the entire fistulous tract is then sharply excised (Fig. 42B).

The electrocautery is used for hemostasis. We leave the wound open and let it heal by granulation. Management of the wound in this way results in a fine, hairline scar. Our reluctance to place sutures is related to the likelihood of entrapment of some bacteria, producing wound infection (Fig. 42C). In our experience, these wounds almost universally heal. It is the very rare patient who needs further surgical debridement. It is also very unusual for a second fistula-in-ano to occur. Cryptotomy is not recommended for other crypts in these patients because of the rarity of a second lesion developing.

Reference

Shafer AD, McGlone TP, Flanagan RA: Abnormal crypts of Morgagni: the cause of perianal abscess and fistula-in-ano. J Pediatr Surg 22:203–204, 1987.

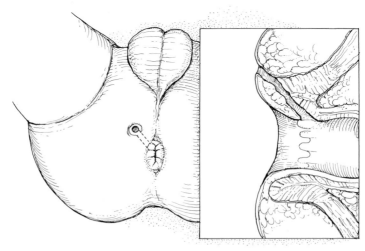

Figure 42A

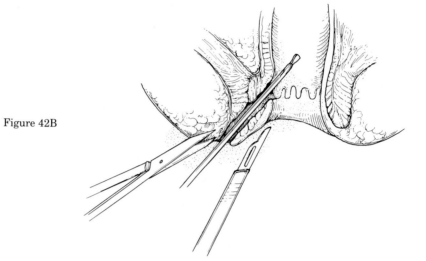

Figure 42B

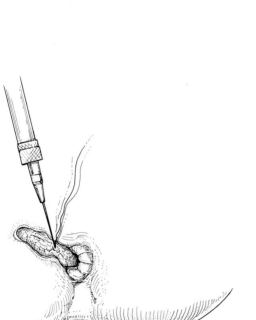

Figure 42C

CHAPTER

43

Endorectal
pull-through

Endorectal pull-through with ileoanal anastomosis is performed most often for ulcerative colitis and familial polyposis. In some patients who have a colectomy for severe ulcerative colitis, a Hartmann's pouch is left for the possible performance of an ileoanal pull-through procedure. This procedure is usually performed in the anabolic state, months or even years after colectomy. In patients with milder forms of ulcerative colitis or polyposis, ileoanal pull-through may be done as a primary procedure at the time of colectomy.

The patient is placed supine on the operative table with the knees over knee crutches so that the abdomen and the anus can both be approached without moving the patient. An indwelling catheter is placed into the urinary bladder and led off under the drape. The abdominal approach may be through a midline vertical or transverse lower abdominal incision depending on whether the colectomy has been done previously or is to be done at the time of the ileoanal pull-through. The pelvis approach is first, and if a Hartmann's pouch is present, a muscular cuff is developed (Fig. 43A). In patients with ulcerative colitis, it may be difficult to develop this plane because of the inflammatory response. Traction on the mucosal tube, with countertraction on the muscular sleeve, and the use of both blunt and sharp dissection as well as electrocautery facilitate this process.

The dissection is carried as far inferiorly from the abdominal approach as possible. It is exceedingly important not to leave mucosal remnants on the inside of the muscular cuff; these may lead to postoperative complications such as cuff abscess or mucocele formation, which will interfere with satisfactory outcome.

Development of the endorectal cuff is completed from below. A circumferential incision is made through the mucosa at the level of the crypts. The dissection proceeds proximally until it meets that from above.

Several techniques are available to create a reservoir that allows the patient to store a little more stool and need to evacuate less often (Fig. 43B). The lateral ileal reservoir is illustrated in which a segment 10 cm long is separated from continuity with the ileum and anastomosed side to side using a stapler, leaving one limb 1.5 cm longer for the anal anastomosis. The upper portion of the lateral ileal reservoir is either stapled or sutured directly to the ileum to make a pouch that has no blind pocket. The distal limb of the reservoir is sutured to the anal skin using absorbable suture material. The pouch should fit within the muscular cuff and should be sutured to it so that retraction will not occur. Alternative reservoirs are the "S"-shaped reservoir illustrated in Figures 43C, 43D, and 43E, and the "J"-shaped reservoir illustrated in Figures 43F, 43G, and 43H. We prefer the lateral ileal or "J" reservoir.

A protective ileostomy should be carried out at the time the reservoir is created, closing over the distal ileum as it comes into the pelvis to form the endorectal pull-through. This will protect the pull-through during its period of healing. A formal laparotomy is required to anastomose the ileum. This should probably be done no earlier than 4 months after creation of the endorectal pull-through.

All patients have frequent loose stools for several months. The major complication is incomplete emptying of the pouch and "pouchitis," often associated with some degree of stenosis. However, most patients feel this is a small price to pay to avoid the permanent ileostomy appliance.

Reference

Fonkalsrud EW: Inflammatory bowel disease. In Ashcraft KW, Holder TM, eds: Pediatric Surgery. 2nd ed. Philadelphia, WB Saunders, 1993, pp 440–452.

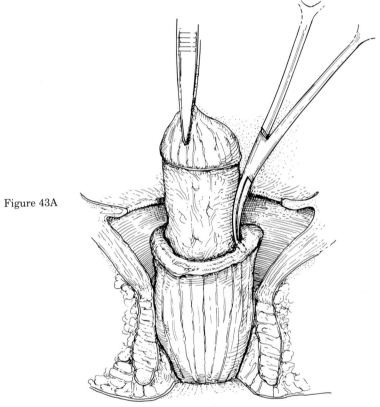

Figure 43A

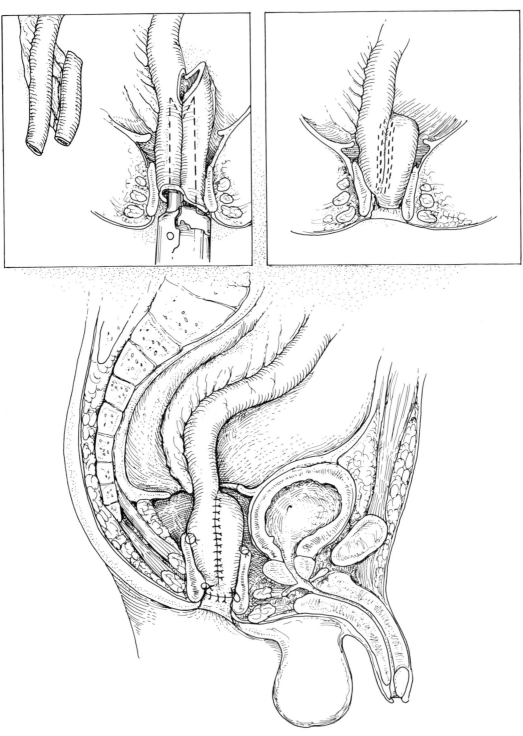

Figure 43B

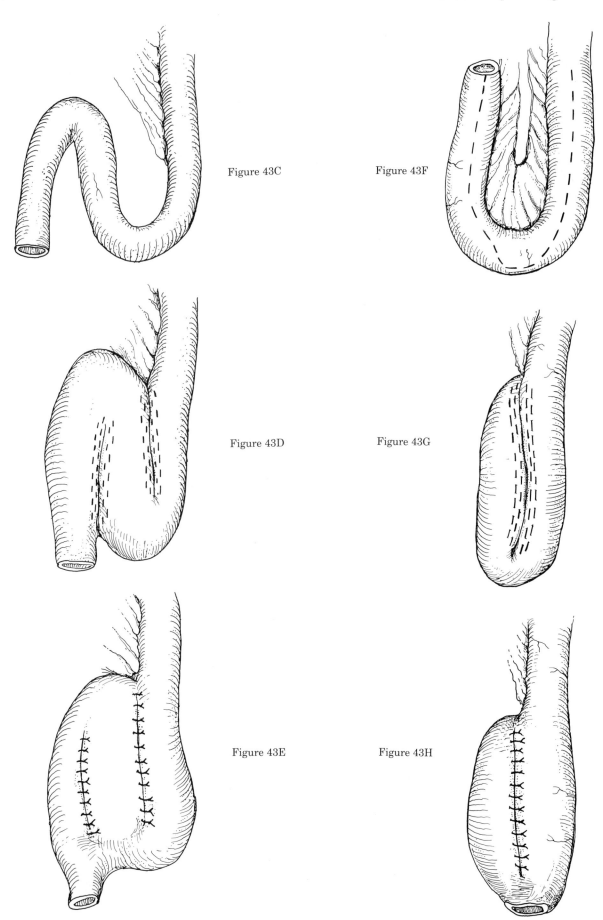

Figure 43C

Figure 43F

Figure 43D

Figure 43G

Figure 43E

Figure 43H

44

Cloaca

The cloaca is a very unusual malformation in the female child in which the rectum, vagina, and urethra come together and exit the body as a single opening between the well-developed labia majora and labia minora. These malformations are often exceedingly complex, with either a bifid vagina, each having its own uterus, or a septate vagina. Part or all of the internal genitalia may be missing. The vagina may be very short, and its satisfactory construction may require the interposition of a segment of colon or small bowel. Urinary tract abnormalities include agenesis of a kidney and vesicoureteric reflux.

These patients require extensive evaluation prior to operative treatment. The operative correction of cloacal malformations often requires combined posterior sagittal and abdominal approaches. The most extensive work in this field has been done by Hendren. The illustrations in this chapter are not intended to be anything other than the most simplistic concept of a cloacal repair.* Prior to an operative case, the reader should consult the references listed.

The operative approach requires that the patient be prepped in such a way that she can be turned from front to back and back again, as is illustrated in Chapter 37 on Hirschsprung's disease. The initial surgical incision is a midline posterior incision (Fig. 44A).

Viewed sagittally, the confluence of the bladder, urethra, vagina, and rectum opens in the perineum anterior to the sphincter mechanism of the rectum. The surgeon's task is to separate these structures so that the urinary tract, the reproductive tract, and the gastrointestinal tract are separate entities in the perineum (Fig. 44B). The approach is the same as that used for the posterior sagittal anorectoplasty. An incision is made in the midline from over the lower portion of the sacrum down to the orifice of the cloaca (Fig. 44C). The muscle complex of the rectum must be identified and labeled. The best way to identify these muscles is to use an electrical stimulator. The muscle complex and the levator muscles are split in the midline and retracted laterally as the incision in the cloaca is carried forward, exposing the rectum, the vaginal opening, and the urethra, which is shown with an indwelling catheter in Figure 44D.

Careful identification of each of these tubular structures is important so that the rectum may be dissected free of the posterior wall of the vagina (Fig. 44E). This is usually done with needlepoint electrocautery, which allows ac-

---

*All figures redrawn from figures in Frank JD, Johnston JH: Operative Paediatric Urology. New York, Churchill Livingstone, 1990.

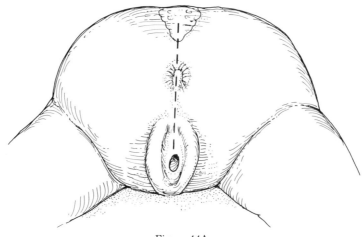

Figure 44A

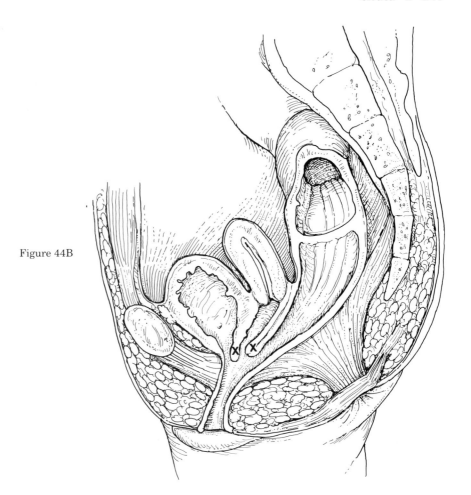

Figure 44B

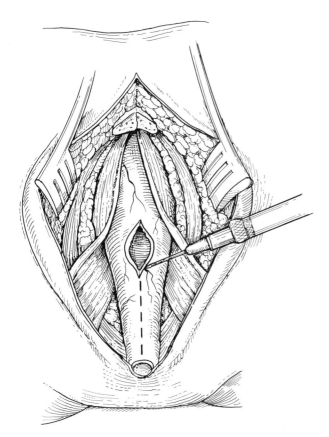

Figure 44C

curate dissection and provides some hemostasis. Lateral traction sutures are placed to allow rapid reidentification of each structure as the perineum is reassembled.

The rectum is freed from the vagina and dissected a reasonable distance cephalad so that the two structures are easily separable. The rectum must reach the neoanus without tension. It is important that intact rectal wall abuts the vagina. It may be necessary to place additional traction sutures both in the end of the rectum and in the posterior wall of the vagina. The vagina is then dissected free of the urethra. The urinary sphincter is located above this point.

The vagina is very carefully dissected free of the posterior portion of the urethra to preserve the urinary sphincter (Fig. 44F).

The urethra is then closed with interrupted or continuous sutures all the way to the cutaneous junction of the cloaca to provide a very long urethra (Fig. 44G).

The vagina is mobilized only as much as necessary to bring it to the perineum, where it is approximated to the labia minora as a separate and distinct orifice from the urethra (Fig. 44H). This approximation should be carried out with absorbable sutures. The fatty tissue and the anterior portion of the muscle complex that form the sphincter mechanism for the anorectum are then brought together with interrupted permanent sutures behind the vagina but anterior to the rectum.

The rectum is trimmed to length and tapered posteriorly, if necessary, for it to fit comfortably within the muscle complex (Fig. 44I). The anal anastomo-

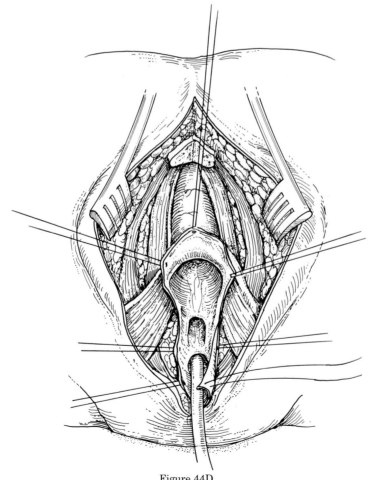

Figure 44D

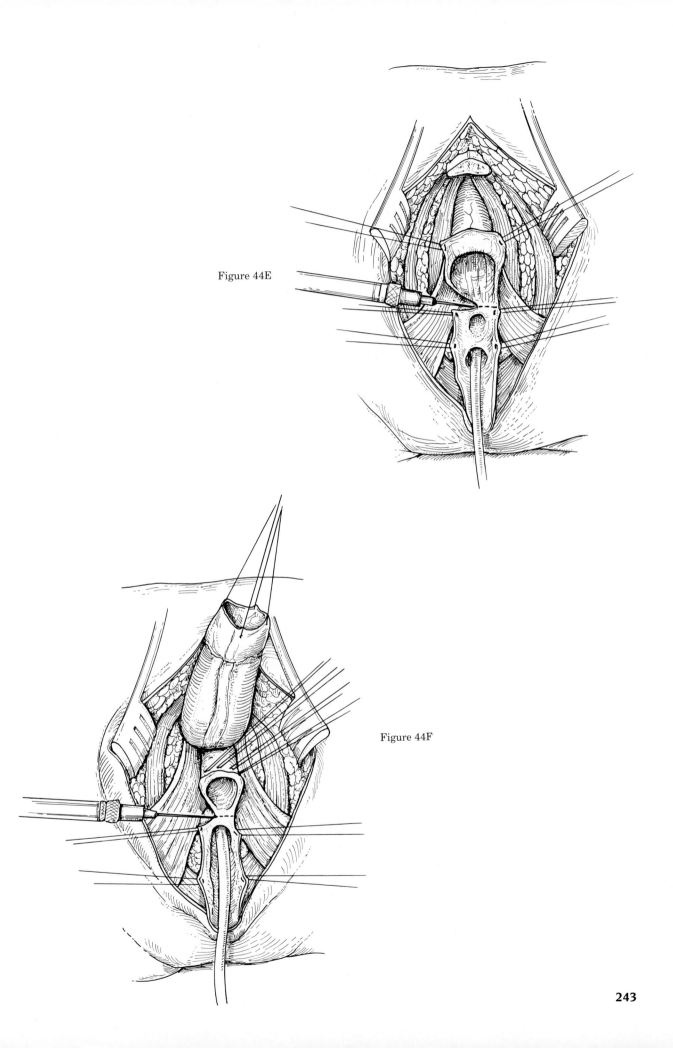

Figure 44E

Figure 44F

sis to the skin is described in the chapter dealing with imperforate anus (Chapter 36). The cutaneous flaps are turned up laterally to reach the rectum, providing an anal canal that is partially lined by perianal skin. The posterior muscle complex is brought together with interrupted permanent sutures to complete the sphincteric and support mechanism for the anorectum. The anastomosis of the anorectum to the skin is carried out with permanent monofilament sutures, which, as in imperforate anus, are removed 2 weeks after the operative procedure. Dilatations of the anorectum are then begun (Fig. 44*I*).

A sagittal view of the corrected cloaca is shown in Figure 44*J*. It is important that the posterior suture line in the newly constructed urethra abut against solid anterior vaginal wall and that tailoring of the vagina be carried out posteriorly, if necessary, so that it abuts against normal pulled-through rectal wall. Tailoring of the rectum and closure of the levator muscle complex behind the rectum are then accomplished. All of these maneuvers minimize the probability of fistula formation.

The completed repair is shown in Figure 44*K*. The perianal sutures and the sutures closing the midline posteriorly are removed at 2 weeks, and anal dilatation is begun. Hegar dilators are used, increasing by one size each week. When the anus has been dilated to No. 12 French in an infant or No. 16 French in a toddler, the colostomy may be closed. To allow healing to occur,

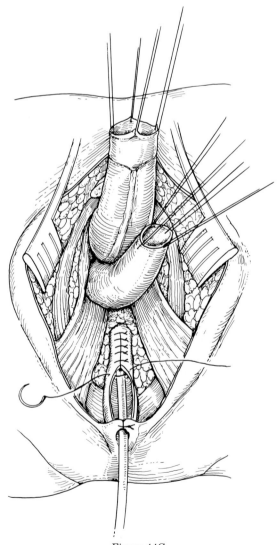

Figure 44G

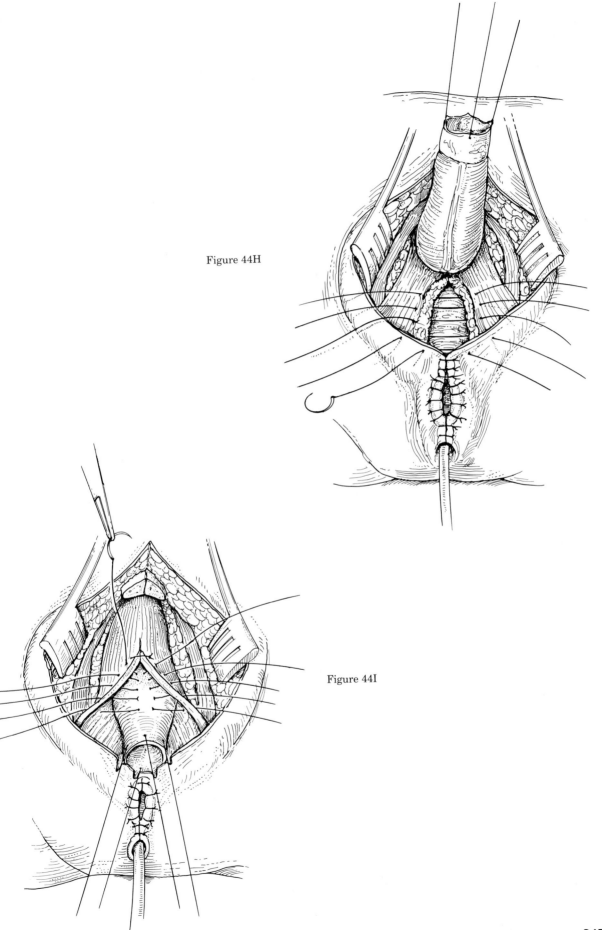

Figure 44H

Figure 44I

dilatation of the urethra and the vaginal opening is not carried out for a protracted period. Therefore, sutures in this area should be absorbable.

Potential complications with repair of cloaca include fistula formation from one hollow viscus to the next, and incontinence of urine and feces owing to inappropriate dissection around the urethral sphincter and inappropriate placement of the rectum through the anal sphincter.

References

Hendren WH: Repair of cloacal anomalies: current techniques. J Pediatr Surg 21:1159–1176, 1986.

Pena A: The surgical management of persistent cloaca: results in 54 patients treated with a posterior sagittal approach. J Pediatr Surg 24:590–598, 1989.

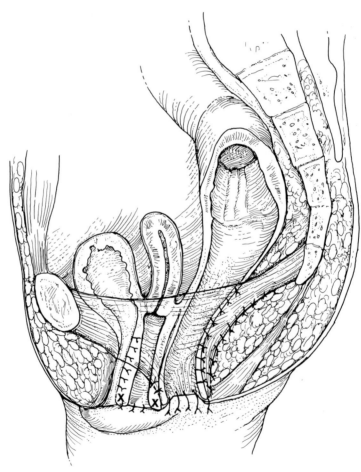

Figure 44J

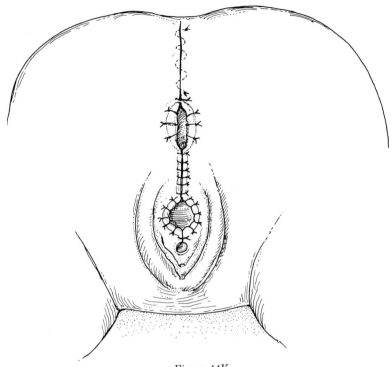

Figure 44K

CHAPTER

45

Inguinal hernia

Inguinal hernia remains the most common operative procedure in pediatric patients other than bilateral myringotomy and placement of tubes for chronic otitis. Indirect inguinal hernias are congenital, tend to be familial, and may present at any age. They are more common in males and may present as a fluid-filled scrotum that changes in size. Fluid around the testicle that persists after 4 to 6 months of age is presumed to be due to a connection with the peritoneal cavity; this communication is a hernia sac. We reserve the term "hydrocele" for the isolated hydrocele often seen in newborns that resolves spontaneously. Hydroceles may also be seen in older patients. They are sometimes inflammatory or may be traumatic, and most often they are self-limiting.

An inguinal hernia in the male may present as a bulge above the inguinal crease and near the base of the penis, or it may extend into the scrotum (Fig. 45A). In the female, protrusion occurs in approximately the same area but sometimes will turn upward so that the lump is felt a little higher (Fig. 45B). The most common organ to occupy a hernia sac in females is the ovary.

The diagnosis of inguinal hernia can be difficult in children and infants, because the sac is not always filled. Palpation of the spermatic cord as it crosses the pubic tubercle is helpful. Rolling the cord under the examining finger will often reveal the "silk glove" sign, which is a slickness or slippage of vas and vessels as the finger is moved back and forth. Experience in palpation of many normal cords will allow differentiation of the cord containing a hernia sac (Fig. 45C). This same "silk glove" sign may be felt in the presence of a lipoma of the cord. Although there are no vas and vessels to slip in the wall of the hernia sac in the female, the physician can often get the same sensation from palpation of the corresponding area in the female.

Protrusion of the intestine in the hernia sac through the internal and external rings constricts the venous outflow of the misplaced viscus, and incarceration occurs as a result of swelling. Strangulation occurs if and when the arterial pressure is exceeded and the process of necrosis begins. Reduction of the hernia is aided by downward pressure of the surgeon's fingers on the abdominal wall to dislodge the overhanging swollen intestine (Fig. 45D). Thus a funnel is created through which pressure on the lower portion of the hernia sac may be directed to restore the viscus to its rightful place within the abdominal cavity. Attempts to reduce the hernia without creating this funnel

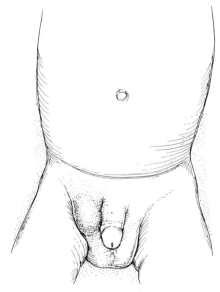

Figure 45A

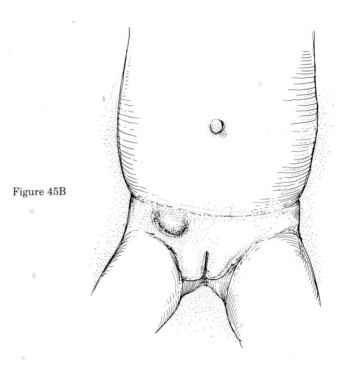

Figure 45B

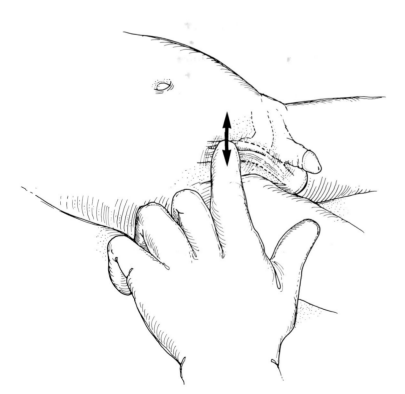

Figure 45C

effect are unlikely to be successful (Fig. 45*D*, inset). Sometimes a good deal of pressure is necessary to return the viscus to the abdominal cavity, but progress can be determined by gradual diminution in either the edema or the content of the entrapped loop of intestine. A hernia that cannot be reduced probably contains seriously compromised bowel, and additional attempts at reduction under anesthesia should be avoided. It is best to explore the patient with the hernia filled so that the involved loop can be easily inspected before its return to the abdominal cavity.

If the surgeon is successful in reducing the hernia, the patient should be scheduled for hernia repair about 48 hours later, which gives the inguinal edema a chance to resolve.

Reduction of an ovary in females is sometimes very difficult, always painful, and often futile, because it will simply "pop out" once again. Because the vascular pedicle to the ovary is very narrow, there is little chance that vascular compromise of this organ will occur, even though the ovary remains in the hernia sac. Plans for elective correction of the hernia are made after reduction.

A controversy exists in pediatric surgery as to the best way to determine whether a hernia is present on the side opposite the side of presentation. Exploration of the opposite side is the simplest way to determine the presence of a hernia sac, and if one is present, it should be removed. We mark the midline (Fig. 45*E*) with a skin marker or place dots or a line on the incision in

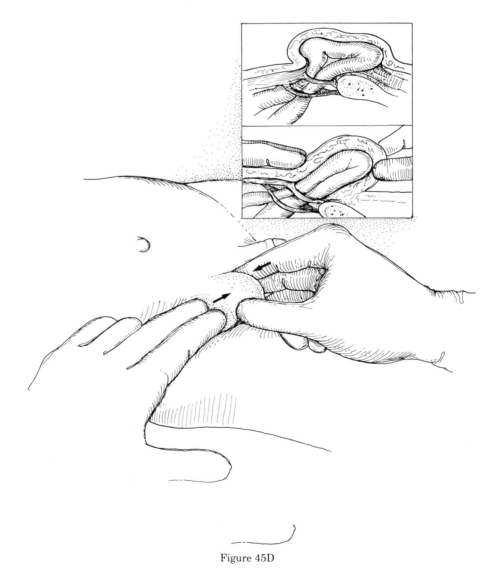

Figure 45D

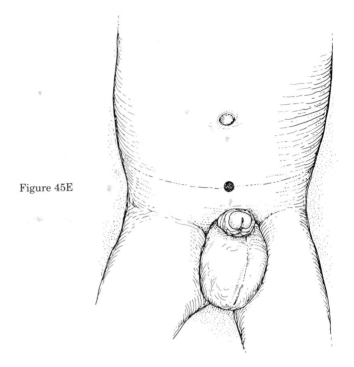

Figure 45E

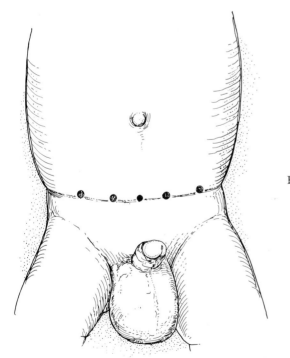

Figure 45F

the inguinal crease on both sides (Fig. 45F) so that symmetry is maintained. Once the patient is prepped and draped, it is sometimes difficult to determine the midline without some marking system.

For postoperative pain control, we use 0.5% bupivacaine hydrochloride (Marcaine) up to a dose of 0.3 ml/kg. About half the dose is injected in the area of the incisions (Fig. 45G). The remaining local anesthetic is injected into the area of the spermatic cord at completion of the procedure. Some surgeons use a caudal block performed by the anesthesiologist either before or after the procedure; this works quite well.

An incision is made in the skin to connect the dots (Fig. 45H). A superficial epigastric vein is often encountered. Two clamps are applied to this vein, and it is divided. The clamps are then used to retract the center portion of the wound so that Scarpa's fascia may be incised and the external oblique aponeurosis exposed. The two veins are then cauterized and the clamps removed (Fig. 45I).

Small "S" retractors are placed medially and inferiorly in the wound to bring the wound down over the external inguinal ring. Scissors are used to clean the external oblique aponeurosis down to this area (Fig. 45J).

A blunt periosteal elevator is then inserted into the external inguinal ring and used to protect the cord structures and the nerve as the external oblique aponeurosis is incised in the direction of its fibers upward and laterally (Fig. 45K). Scarpa's fascia needs to be incised for only 1½ to 2 cm. The external oblique aponeurosis is then cleaned off of the cord, the cord grasped, and the cremaster fibers separated so that the sac can be lifted. The vas and the vessels are carefully dissected from the underside of the arch formed by tenting the sac (Fig. 45L).

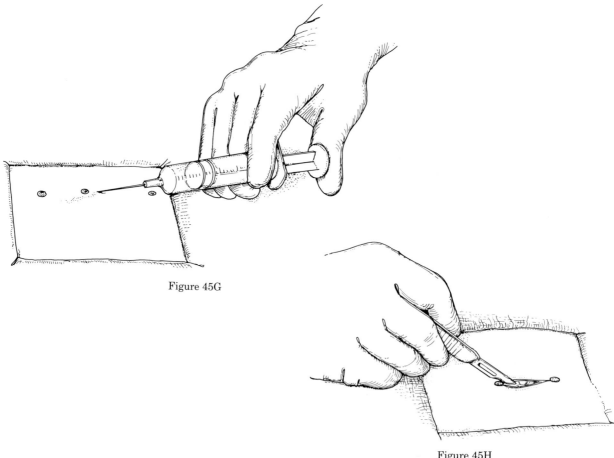

Figure 45G

Figure 45H

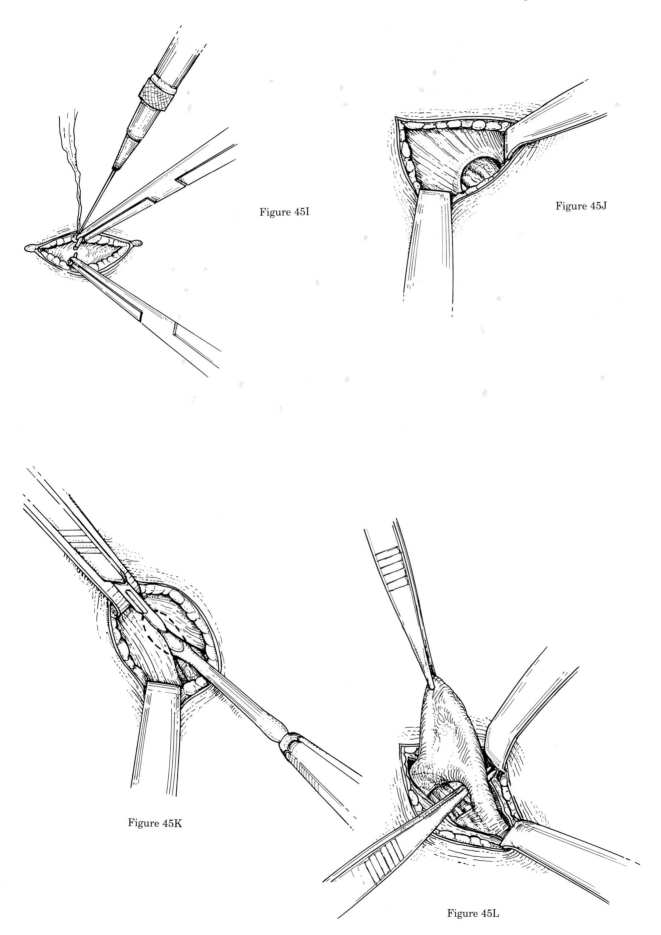

Figure 45I

Figure 45J

Figure 45K

Figure 45L

A straight hemostat inserted between the sac and the cord structures is spread to further dissect the vas and the vessels away from a length of sac (Fig. 45M). Two straight hemostats are then used to clamp the sac, which is then divided (Fig. 45N).

The proximal sac is dissected up to the internal inguinal ring, taking the vas and vessels off in a manner designed to protect them from injury (Fig. 45O). Any crush injury to the vas with tissue forceps or a clamp will probably result in luminal obstruction by scar.

Suture ligation of the sac, with a permanent suture placed at the peritoneal level, is then accomplished. The proximal sac is trimmed, leaving a stump long enough that it does not slip through the suture ligature (Fig. 45P).

The distal hernia sac is then dissected. Often it will be found to be continuous with the tunica vaginalis. Great care must be taken at this point to avoid injury to the vas deferens or the epididymis, which is sometimes splayed out over the surface of the sac and is therefore liable to injury. Because the epididymis is a continuous single tube, an interruption at any point is considered to be a permanent division of the spermatic duct (Fig. 45Q). However, there have been reports of epididymal structures in the wall of the sac that are not connected to the spermatic duct.

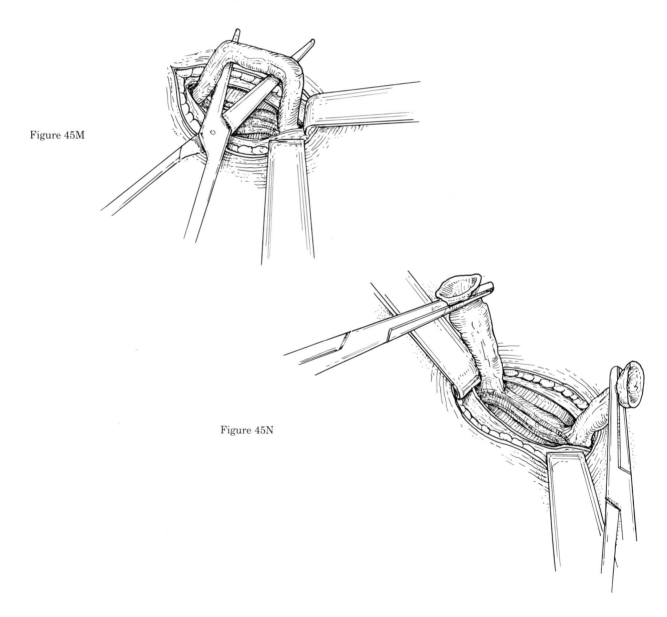

Figure 45M

Figure 45N

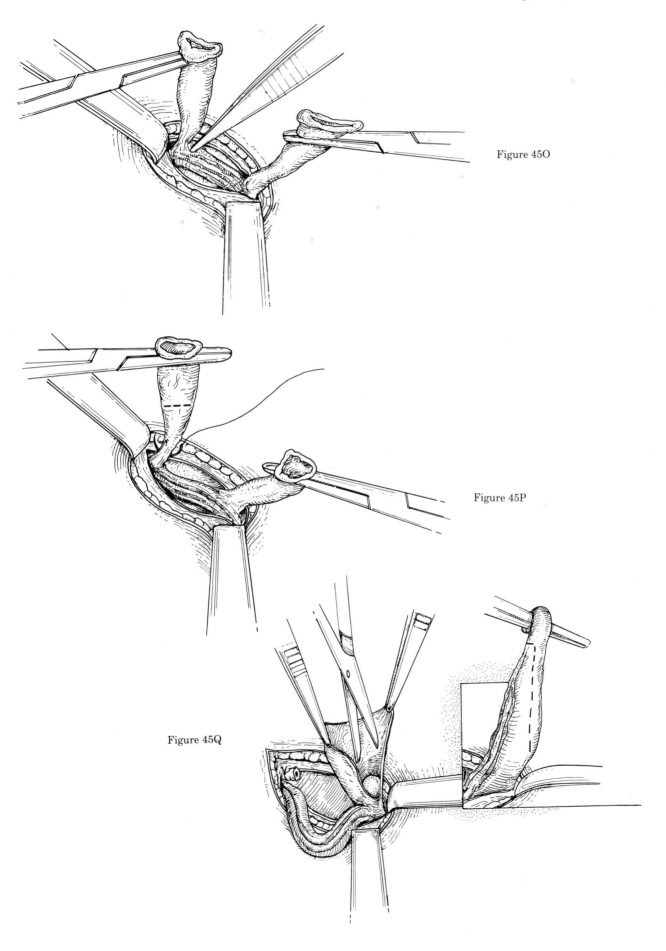

Figure 45O

Figure 45P

Figure 45Q

In our technique, the testicle is delivered back into the scrotum by inserting a blunt periosteal elevator (joker elevator) into the tunica vaginalis and pushing the testicle downward into the scrotum (Fig. 45R). Alternatively, if the scrotum has been prepped, it may be grasped and stretched downward, which will deliver the testicle back into the scrotum.

Children rarely require repair of the internal inguinal ring. If such repair is necessary, this is done by lifting the cord structures off the inguinal floor and placing permanent sutures of appropriate-size silk in a figure-of-8 fashion to narrow the ring (Fig. 45S). It is even more rare that a child will require Cooper's ligament repair, but if this is necessary, it is done in the same manner used in an adult.

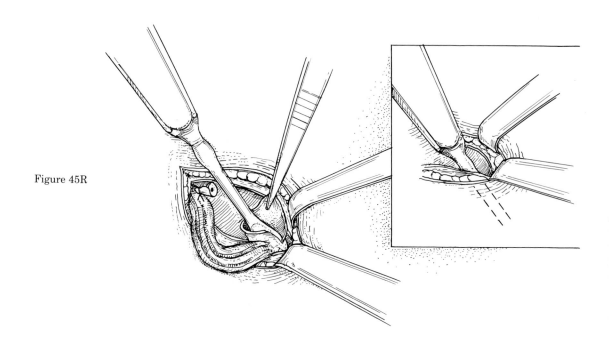

Figure 45R

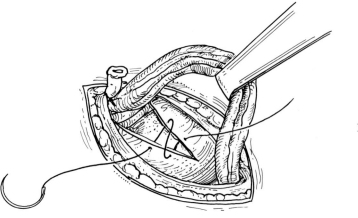

Figure 45S

Once the posterior floor is sutured so that the internal ring is tight but not strangulating the cord (Fig. 45T), the hernia repair is complete.

The external oblique aponeurosis is reapproximated (Fig. 45U), and a small amount of bupivacaine hydrochloride is injected through the fascia into the area of the cord. This provides additional pain relief for the patient during the postoperative period.

Scarpa's fascia is approximated loosely and the skin sutured with subcuticular absorbable (Dexon) sutures (Fig. 45V). Appropriate dressings include flexible collodion for the infant in diapers and Steri-Strips for the toilet-trained child. After wound closure, the testes are checked to ensure that they are in the scrotum (Fig. 45W). If they are not and cannot be manipulated into the scrotum, it will be necessary to prep the patient again, open the wound, and place the testicle in its proper position.

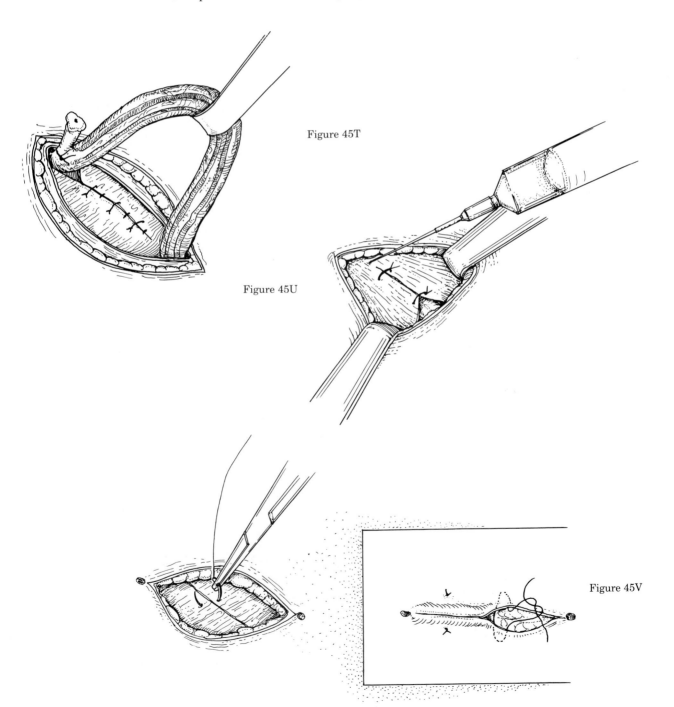

Figure 45T

Figure 45U

Figure 45V

The completed operative procedure in the male is shown in Figure 45X.

In the female, the entire sac is dissected from the inguinal canal. It often will contain suspensory ligaments from the ovary or the fallopian tube itself. The hernia may be managed by opening the sac and placing a pursestring suture just distal to the attachments of the ovary so that as this pursestring is tied, the ovary and its appendages are isolated to the peritoneal cavity (Fig. 45Y).

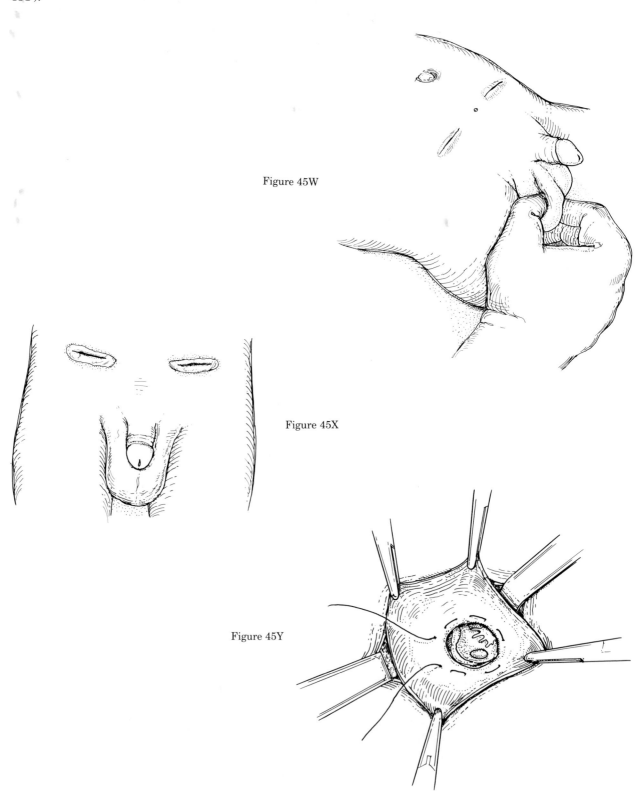

Figure 45W

Figure 45X

Figure 45Y

Alternatively, the sac may be opened and the attachments of the ovary taken down from inside with an electrocautery (Fig. 45Z). The sac is then twisted and suture ligated (Fig. 45AA) to complete the hernia repair.

In our experience, the hernia recurrence rate is about 1 per 1000 cases. Recurrences are more common after herniorrhaphies in premature infants and in those operated on after an episode of incarceration. Injury to the spermatic ducts can also occur; this is a disaster, as the ducts cannot be reliably reconstructed. Great care is urged in dissecting the distal hernia sac because of the possibility of interrupting the epididymis as it is splayed out over a very tense distal hernia sac. The vas, of course, must never be picked up or crushed, because it is believed that a mucosal stricture is very likely to result.

Differentiation of recurrent hernia from recurrent collection of fluid in the scrotum is sometimes difficult. The impression of fluctuation in size is produced by contraction of the scrotal skin, and therefore, the only sure way to demonstrate recurrent hernia is with a herniogram (i.e., injection of contrast material into the peritoneal cavity while holding the infant upright). This is an uncomfortable procedure and one that is not without risk of inflammatory adhesions because of the contrast material. Leaving a generous amount of distal sac to avoid epididymal injury may result in postoperative secretion of fluid. We often aspirate such a collection several times to avoid the necessity for a herniogram.

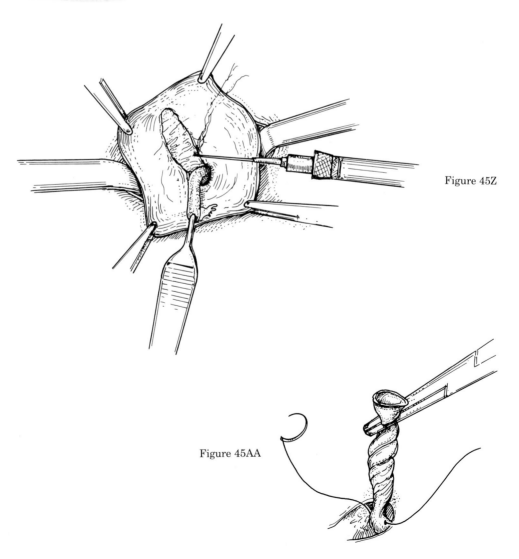

Figure 45Z

Figure 45AA

Umbilical hernia

Umbilical hernias are common defects in children, particularly black children. They are reputed to close spontaneously in about 90% to 95% of cases, but the actual incidence of spontaneous closure is impossible to estimate.

In our experience, two forms of umbilical hernia exist. The first consists of those very grotesque hernias associated with a protuberance of skin, on the end of which is an umbilicus. Regardless of the size of the fascial defect, spontaneous healing of these umbilical hernias will leave the patient with a very unsatisfactory abdominal wall and a great deal of excessive skin. Although most of the defects are large, they sometimes have a diameter smaller than that of a fingertip (Fig. 46A).

The other kind of umbilical hernia is one that has a much less protuberant bit of skin associated with it (Fig. 46B). The fascial defect may or may not be large. Many times, if followed over a period of time, these fascial defects will be seen to reduce in size. If the patient is asymptomatic and will not be left with an unsightly umbilicus after spontaneous closure, we elect to perform repair after the age of 3 years.

In patients with grotesque umbilical hernias (Fig. 46C), we elect to perform repair at almost any age, even in the first 6 months of life. When performing an umbilicoplasty in these patients, we prefer to make a circumferential incision very near the base of the umbilical sac and remove both the protuberance of skin and the sac. The ensuing fascial defect (Fig. 46D) is closed in a transverse manner (Fig. 46E) using figure-of-8 sutures of 2-0 or 3-0 Gore-Tex. Gore-Tex is exceedingly strong and very soft and will not leave palpable knots beneath the subcutaneous tissue as occur with some of the monofilament permanent suture materials. The umbilicoplasty is accomplished with an absorbable continuous pursestring suture (Fig. 46F), which puckers the umbilicus and forms a very stellate umbilicus. This is not normal, but it has a much more normal appearance than does the umbilicus with a large amount of skin.

In patients with an umbilical hernia without grotesque skin involvement, a smiling incision is made within the umbilical substance itself (Fig. 46G), and the skin is dissected free of the umbilical hernia sac. The hernia sac is circumcised at the fascial level and may be either tucked in or removed (Fig. 46H). The same transverse closure using figure-of-8 Gore-Tex sutures is performed (Fig. 46E). Subcuticular sutures are used to reapproximate the skin beneath the umbilicus (Fig. 46I), and the standard asterisk dressing using ½-inch × 4-inch Steri-Strips is applied (Fig. 46J). The Steri-Strip dressing is applied so that loose umbilical skin is pressed down against the abdominal wall. Because exertion forces the abdominal wall up against the umbilical skin, the Steri-Strips are left in place for as long as they will stay. This has proved to be a very satisfactory pressure dressing device and obviates the skin shear that frequently occurs with Elastoplast dressings.

Recurrence of umbilical hernias after using Gore-Tex sutures has been very rare. Infection has been virtually eliminated in our experience.

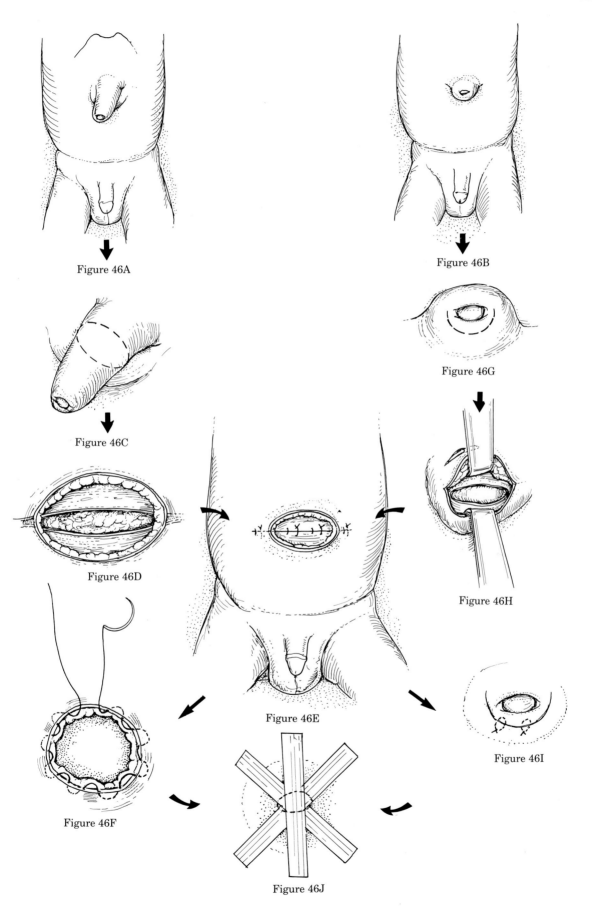

Figure 46A

Figure 46B

Figure 46C

Figure 46G

Figure 46D

Figure 46H

Figure 46E

Figure 46F

Figure 46I

Figure 46J

47

Orchiopexy

Undescended testes (UDTs) are a very common occurrence in boys. The testes normally descend in the seventh fetal month, not by traction from the gubernaculum, but by growing down into the substance of the gubernaculum. This process is most often interrupted because the testis is caught within a hernia sac; in fact, 95% of UDTs are associated with inguinal hernia. Operatively manipulated descent of the testes requires division of the hernia sac, which is usually enough to allow the testis to reach to the scrotum without further dissection. Of course, repair of the hernia is accomplished at the same time. The tunica or distal sac is left about the testis as it is delivered down into the scrotum and surgically fixed.

Misdiagnosis of UDT most often occurs when the examiner confuses retractile testes with those that are truly undescended. For this reason, the myth still remains that testes will sometimes spontaneously descend in boys who have not been born prematurely. However, truly undescended testes do not descend without some intervention. Treatment of undescended testes with gonadotropin-releasing hormone (Gn-RH) is more popular in other parts of the world than in the United States. Such treatment is primarily effective when retractile testes are mistaken for undescended testes. Undescended nonpalpable testes may be made palpable by hormonal therapy, but an anatomic hernia that limits the descent of the testes is unlikely to be cured by administration of hormones.

The testes may also be ectopically located (Fig. 47A). Ectopic testes are usually in the medial upper thigh or behind the scrotum. Truly undescended testes may be in the canal at the level of the internal inguinal ring or behind the bladder. The vas is usually not the limiting factor in the descent of the testes. The vas seems to grow to its normal length regardless of the position of the testes, but the arterial supply to the testis will grow only as long as necessary. Usually the length of the artery limits the ability to surgically place the testis within the scrotum.

The approach to an undescended testis is through the standard groin hernia incision. The patient is usually placed supine with the knees apart in

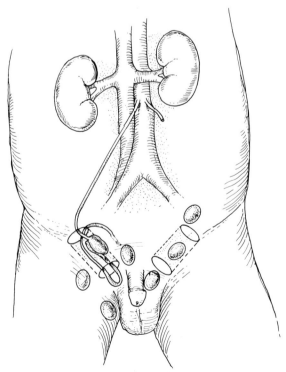

Figure 47A

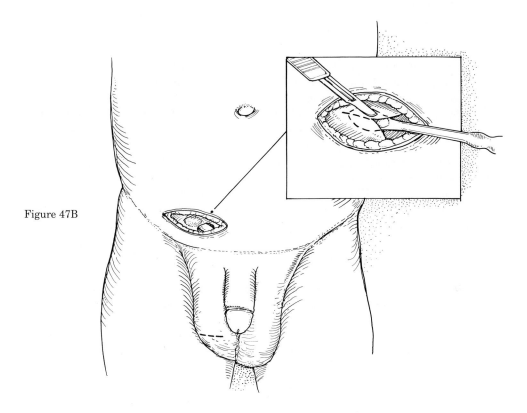

Figure 47B

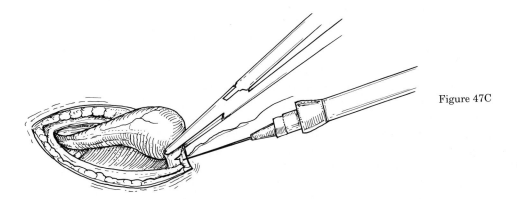

Figure 47C

the "frog-leg" position. We usually drape the patient with three towels, one across the abdomen and one down either groin to meet beneath the scrotum. The lower abdomen and genitalia are all prepped into the surgical field (Fig. 47B). The external oblique aponeurosis is opened as for a hernia incision (Fig. 47B, inset).

Exploration for UDT may reveal the presence of the spermatic cord in the canal, and tracing the cord toward the scrotum will reveal atrophy or dysplasia of the testes. In these circumstances, the testes should be removed, as they are dysplastic and are likely to undergo malignant degeneration later in life. This is true of dysplastic testes regardless of their location. If nothing is found in the inguinal canal, then the testis is usually located within the peritoneal cavity, and exploration must be carried out. In those patients without palpable testes, laparoscopic visualization of the testicular position may be combined with surgical clipping of the spermatic artery so that later, surgically manipulated descent may be accomplished, basing the testis on the newly developed collateral blood supply through the vessels of the vas deferens. Nonpalpable testes occur in less than 1% of patients in our experience.

The majority of UDTs are located within a hernia sac (Fig. 47C). The distal attachments of the hernia sac are divided, and the entire sac is delivered up into the wound and dissected to the level of the internal ring.

The spermatic cord appears to be surrounded entirely by the hernia sac, but there is a point at which the sides of the sac meet (Fig. 47D). The intact hernia sac can be dissected free of cord structures. We prefer to do this dissection at about mid-cord level, very carefully dissecting the sac free of the vas and vessels, isolating the vas and vessels, and then dividing the hernia sac.

The hernia sac is then separated from the cord structures up to the level of the internal ring (Fig. 47E), where it is suture ligated and further trimmed. In most instances the testis within its tunica is then able to reach the scrotum so that little or no additional dissection of the cord is necessary.

If the cord length is not sufficient to allow the testis to be delivered into the scrotum, two maneuvers may be used to improve the situation. Retroperitoneal dissection of the spermatic artery may be accomplished through the internal inguinal ring. If this is not sufficient, the floor of the inguinal canal may be incised to the pubic tubercle, dividing the inferior epigastric vessels (Fig. 47F). These two maneuvers will provide the maximal arterial length and shorten the distance that the artery must travel to allow the testis to reach the scrotum. Undue tension on the testis using traction devices will result in arterial spasm and often in loss of the testis. If no amount of dissection allows the testis to reach the scrotum, then a decision must be made as to whether to remove the testis. It is possible that an undescended testis may ultimately interfere with sperm production on the opposite normal side. It is certainly true that a male with one normally descended testis is statistically about as fertile as a male with two normal testes. Attempts at microvascular testicular autotransplantation or Fowler-Stephens mobilization of the testis by acutely dividing the spermatic artery both have allowed satisfactory relocation of the testes in the scrotum. Most patients undergoing testicular artery division have had insufficient collateral to prevent ultimate loss of the testis.

Scrotal fixation of the mobilized testis requires that a canal to the scrotum be developed. We prefer to create this tunnel with a large Péan clamp (Fig. 47G). Either this large clamp or a finger can be inserted into the scrotum, around which a dartos pouch is developed. A skin incision is made in the scrotum, and blunt dissection with a fine-tipped hemostat is used to separate scrotal skin from dartos fascia (Fig. 47H).

The testis is then delivered on the end of a traction suture, down through an opening in the dartos pouch (Fig. 47I).

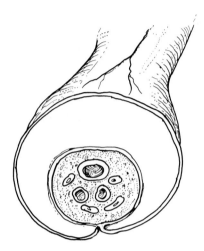

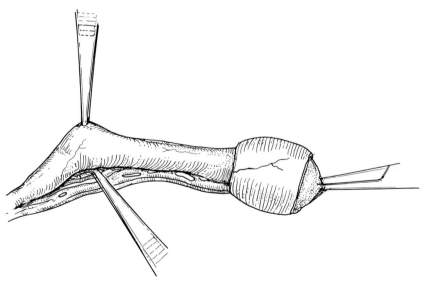

Figure 47D

The cord or the proximal end of the tunica is then attached to the opening of the dartos pouch, creating a testis between the dartos and the skin of the scrotum (Fig. 47*J,* inset). The skin of the scrotum is closed with interrupted or continuous absorbable suture, and then the hernia wound is closed, completing the procedure.

We usually request that the boys stay off straddling toys for the first 3 weeks postoperatively. The success rate with this procedure approaches 99%; the testis remains in the scrotum and grows with its normally descended counterpart.

Bilateral undescended testes are usually operated on one at a time. If, after 6 months, the first operated testis is growing well, we surgically repair the testis on the opposite side.

References

Hadziselimovic F, Herzog B, Seguchi H: Surgical correction of cryptorchidism at two years: electron microscopic and morphometric investigations. J Pediatr Surg 10:19–26, 1975.

Mengel W, Zimmerman FA: Immunologic aspects of cryptorchidism. In Fonkalsrud EW, Mengel W, eds: The Undescended Testis. Chicago, Year Book Medical, 1981, pp 184–194.

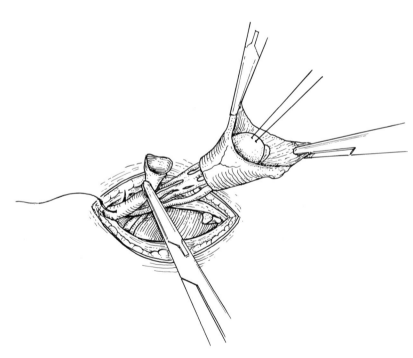

Figure 47E

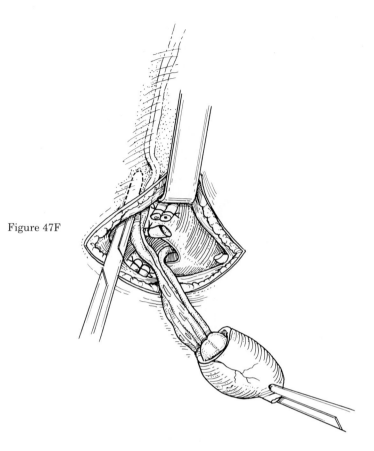

Figure 47F

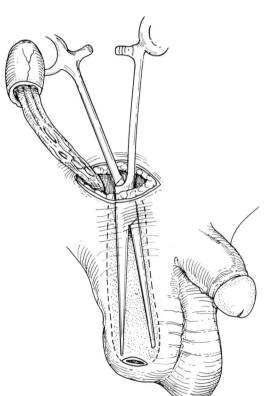

Figure 47G

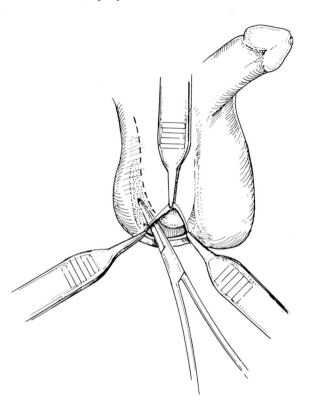

Figure 47H

Figure 47I

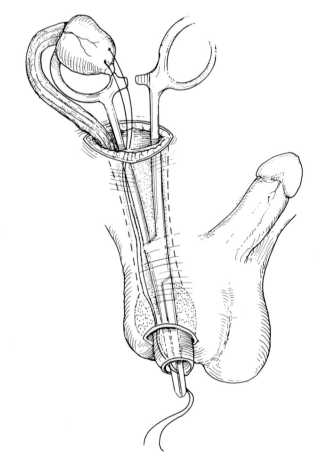

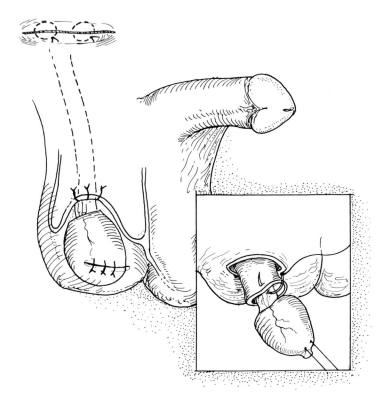

Figure 47J

CHAPTER

48

Wilms' tumor

Wilms' tumor remains a common malignancy in pediatric patients. It is frequently discovered serendipitously by parents during play with the child or by the pediatrician during a routine examination. Wilms' tumors usually present as a large mass that occasionally extends across the midline and well down toward the pelvis. It is often irregular in shape and is not movable. Sometimes the patient will present with hematuria. A normal childhood fall or tumble may result in hemorrhage into the tumor, producing rapid enlargement or hematuria.

Before the operative procedure, a computed tomographic (CT) scan of the entire chest and abdomen should be obtained using contrast material. Wilms' tumor most often metastasizes to the lungs but frequently grows by direct extension into the diaphragm or the liver. A radiograph of the abdomen taken after the CT scan gives one view of an intravenous pyelogram (IVP), which is always helpful in the diagnosis and management of renal fossa tumors. A Wilms' tumor distorts the kidney without displacing it, thereby differentiating it from a neuroblastoma, which most often displaces the kidney without distorting its architecture. Radiographic evidence of lack of function on the side of the tumor suggests that a renal vein tumor thrombus or extension has developed. Conversely, radiographic evidence of normal function indicates that renal vein tumor thrombus is very unlikely to be present.

We prefer to approach removal of these tumors by a transverse upper abdominal incision at the level of the lowest portion of the rib cage. This incision may be extended well around into the flanks to allow wide access to resection of the Wilms' tumor (Fig. 48A).

The tumor is often large, extending across the midline. It will lift the colon and duodenum from their normal positions, but it is rarely intimately attached to the intestine. Periaortic nodes are quite common and should be removed with the tumor (Fig. 48B).

The first step in the operative treatment of a patient with Wilms' tumor is to inspect the opposite kidney. Approximately 5% of patients have coincident Wilms' tumor on the opposite side. Although this is usually easily detectable on the CT scan, it is still worthwhile to open Gerota's fascia on the normal

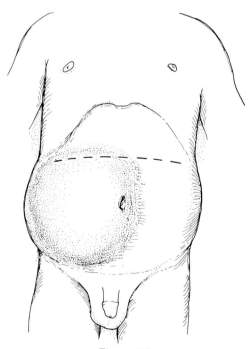

Figure 48A

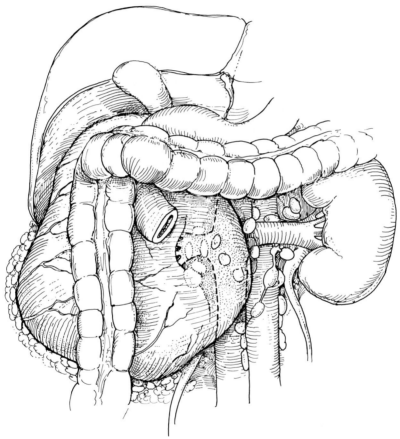

Figure 48B

side and mobilize the kidney entirely, observing its anterior and posterior surfaces and palpating for nodules (Fig. 48C). Wilms' tumor nodules appear yellow or gray and are much firmer than normal kidney tissue. Extensive involvement of both kidneys requires biopsy. Preoperative chemotherapy or radiation is followed by subtotal nephrectomy on one or both sides.

Ninety-five percent of Wilms' tumors are unilateral. The colon should be reflected off the tumor, allowing access to the aorta and inferior vena cava as well as the renal vessels (Fig. 48D). The adrenal gland should be left attached to the kidney and submitted to the pathologist as part of the tumor specimen. Often there are large tumor vessels on the surface of the Wilms' tumor. It is important to achieve good hemostasis with electrocautery or suture ligature. Care must be taken, as it is possible to rupture the capsule or pseudocapsule of the tumor and spill tumor cells throughout the abdominal cavity. Although chemotherapy is usually very effective, tumor spill statistically reduces the chances of the patient's survival. Depending on the size of the tumor, it may not be possible to expose the renal artery and vein initially to divide them, but as with extirpation of any major organ, it is probably best to divide arterial and venous blood vessels to the organ before extensive mobilization.

The renal vein will be the most superficial vessel and should be palpated to determine whether tumor thrombus has propagated within this vascular structure (Fig. 48E, inset). If it has not, it can be mobilized, gaining control of the renal artery. It is probably best to suture ligate or doubly ligate the renal artery proximally and distally before division. The vein is similarly managed before division. After these vessels are divided, the kidney may be mobilized with less blood loss (Fig. 48E).

If tumor thrombus extends into the vena cava, it must be determined, if possible, how far up toward the heart this tumor thrombus extends. The CT scan generally produces evidence of tumor thrombus, and thus this should not come as a surprise to the surgeon. If, indeed, there is tumor thrombus in the renal vein that extends into the lumen of the cava but not up to the level of the diaphragm, then snares are passed about the inferior vena cava, above and below the renal vein, and on the renal vein on the opposite side (Fig. 48F). The involved vein may then be opened and the tumor thrombus removed. The snares prevent exsanguinating hemorrhage, but there will be bleeding from lumbar veins entering the vena cava. The incision in the vena cava or the orifice of the involved renal vein may then be closed with a continuous permanent suture and the tourniquets released, re-establishing caval flow (Fig. 48F, inset).

The specimen is then removed (Fig. 48G), dividing the ureter as low in the operative field as can be easily reached. Attachments to the diaphragm and the liver may need to be divided with cautery, attempting to take as little normal tissue as necessary. Remnants of tumor may have to be left if there is extensive invasion of the liver or the diaphragm, but in our experience, this does not reduce the survival rate of patients with Wilms' tumor if histologic analysis is favorable.

Adjunctive treatment includes a number of chemotherapy protocols designed by the National Wilms' Tumor Study Group. Postoperative radiation of the renal fossa may be used. If chemotherapy is not effective in relieving pulmonary metastases, then surgery may be worthwhile.

Postoperative complications generally include adhesive small bowel obstruction and sometimes recurrent tumor. The outlook for these children is usually dependent more on the tumor's histologic type than on the completeness of surgical excision. Great strides have been made in the treatment of Wilms' tumor, taking it from a lesion that was invariably fatal in 1940 to one that currently has a survival rate of approximately 95%.

Reference

D'Angio GJ, Breslow N, Beckwith JB, et al: Treatment of Wilms' tumor—results of the Third National Wilms' Tumor Study. Cancer 64:349–360, 1989.

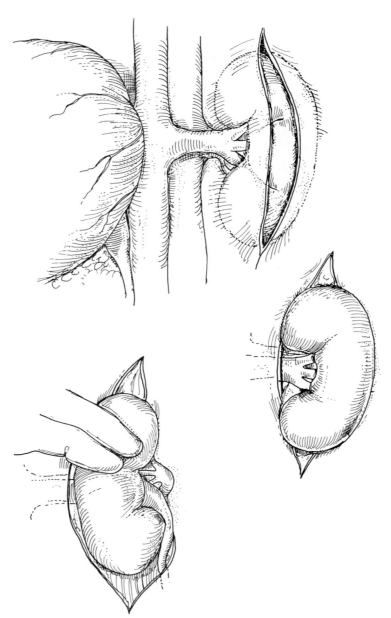

Figure 48C

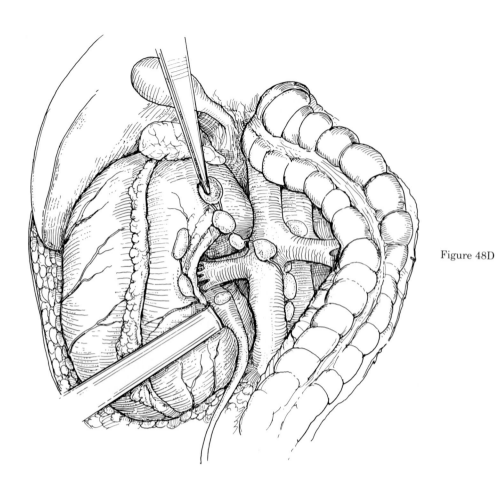

Figure 48D

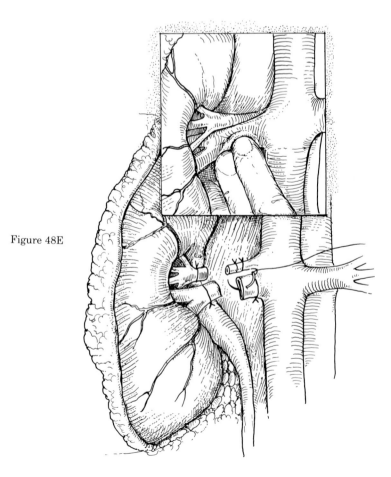

Figure 48E

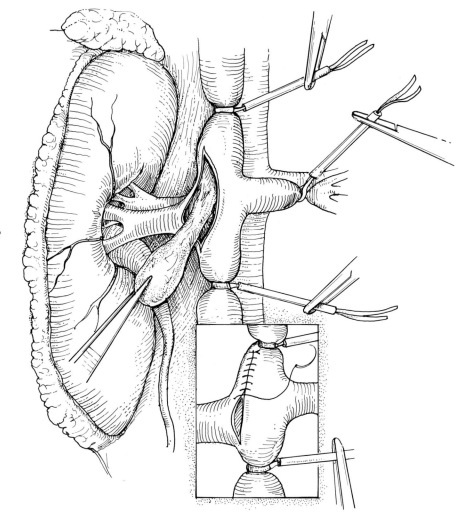

Figure 48F

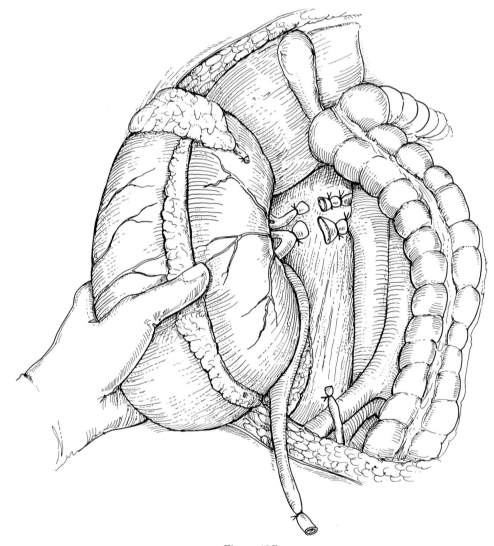

Figure 48G

CHAPTER

49

The acute scrotum

Development of acute pain in the scrotum is a surgical emergency of the first order. Although the pain may be caused by epididymitis or torsion of either the appendix testis or appendix epididymis, it may also be caused by torsion of the testis itself, which, if not promptly reduced, will result in loss of the testis. Usually a careful physical examination is all that is needed to differentiate among these various possibilities. Many times, however, having been seen in the emergency department before the surgeon's examination, the patient will have undergone Doppler ultrasound to determine blood supply to the scrotum, as well as isotope scans, some of which are occasionally helpful.

Torsion of the testis (Fig. 49A) most commonly occurs because the testis is not properly fixed within the tunica and is hanging by only the spermatic cord (the so-called "bell clapper" deformity). Testicular torsion usually occurs in adolescents and usually follows some form of relatively violent exercise. Its onset is acute. The young male is usually reluctant to mention it for several hours until the pain becomes unbearable. If the condition remains unreduced for more than 24 hours, it is rare that the testis can be salvaged. However, if it is reduced in the first 8 hours, it is rare for the testis to be lost. Testicular torsion may occur at any age. In the newborn it is rarely discovered in time to salvage the testis.

A number of small appendages are also present within the scrotum. These small, teardrop-shaped structures attach to the testes, the epididymis, or the distal cord (Fig. 49B) and can twist spontaneously, producing immediate symptoms. These appendages occur most commonly in boys before adolescence. They can often be diagnosed by palpation of a very tender, small mass within the scrotum, in addition to nontender testes and epididymitis. Sometimes a "blue dot" may be apparent through the scrotal skin. Torsion of the appendix testis is followed by spontaneous resorption of the infarcted appendage in about 50% of boys; pain may be relieved by the use of aspirin, acetaminophen (Tylenol), or acetaminophen with codeine for several days. In the other 50%, persistent pain will require surgical removal. It is difficult to predict at the initial visit which boys will require operation, so we usually try nonoperative therapy for several days.

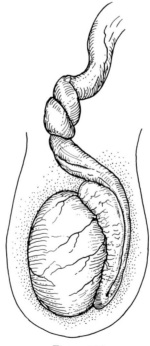

Figure 49A

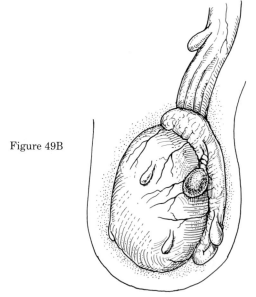

Figure 49B

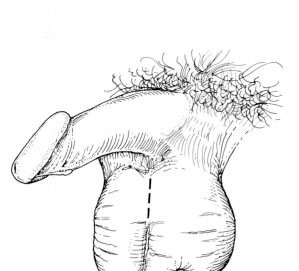

Figure 49C

In the patient who has torsion of the testis, physical examination will reveal a very tender testis, epididymitis, and often a puckering at the lower end of the scrotum (Fig. 49C). The testis and epididymis will be remarkably firm because of venous engorgement and edema. In the case of epididymitis, the testis itself will be soft, but the epididymis will seem boggy and very tender. It is usually not difficult to differentiate epididymitis from torsion of the testis, but if any question exists, the safest method of management is scrotal exploration. This is done through a midline scrotal incision with the patient under general anesthesia. The scrotum is prepped with the penis turned upward and out of the field. A relatively small incision in the midline of the scrotum can be stretched with retractors to allow easy access to the scrotal contents. The incision is deepened off to the involved side, and the tunica is opened with an electrocautery. On approaching the tunica, it is usually obvious that the testis is blue-black. The tunica is opened, and the testis is delivered and untwisted. If there is any evidence of returning color and the testis has been torsed less than 24 hours, it is worthwhile to observe the testis in the operating room for evidence of viability. A small incision in the tunica of the testis will sometimes reveal arterial bleeding, which may indicate that the testis is still viable. Most of the time, however, the testis will not be salvageable unless the patient has presented very early. Therefore, it should be removed, suture ligating the cord at the upper portion of the tunica (Fig. 49D). The removal of an obviously dead testis is important, because such a testis will have no hormonal or reproductive function. There is some evidence that an in situ dead testis may even prevent the normal testicle from producing sperm.

Operative attention is then turned to the opposite, untorsed testis. Assuming that the anatomy of incomplete fixation of the testis is present on the opposite side, the tunica on that side should be opened and the testis examined. If, indeed, this is the case, the tunica is then closed, using interrupted permanent sutures taken also through the tunica covering the testis to produce permanent fixation and prevent torsion on that side (Fig. 49E). Thus, the patient will have one viable testis that is unlikely to undergo torsion.

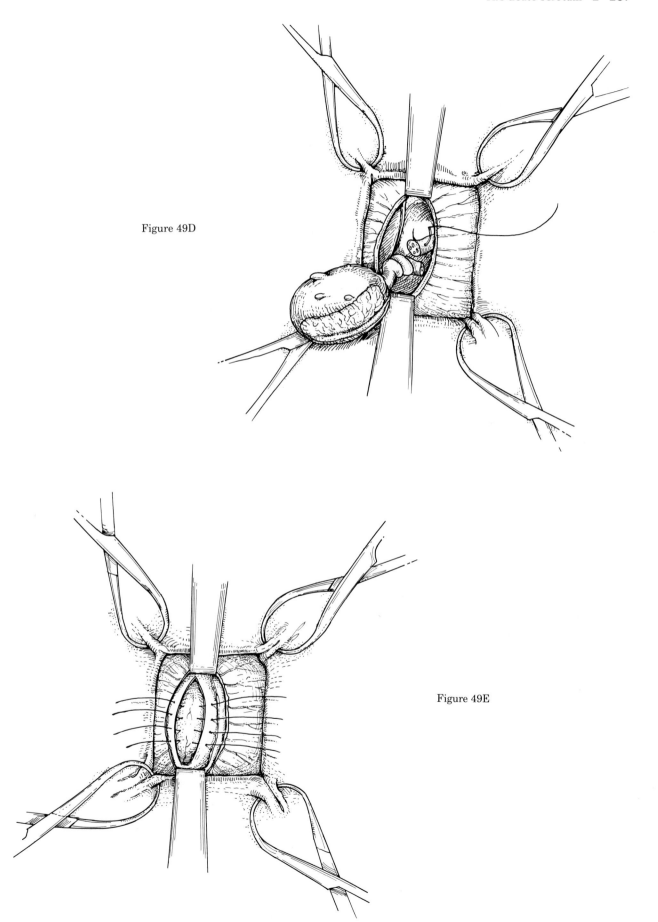

Figure 49D

Figure 49E

50

Duckett urethroplasty

Hypospadias is one of the most common congenital abnormalities in males, reportedly occurring in 1 in every 300 male children.

Normal development of the urethra in its most simple form requires several things to occur at a very sensitive time in the male child's fetal life. Between 7 and 11 weeks of gestation, testosterone must be present in sufficient amounts. The enzyme 5-alpha-reductase is necessary to transform testosterone to dihydrotestosterone, which is the form of the hormone that acts on tissues. In addition, the tissues must be responsive to dihydrotestosterone. Deficiencies in any or all of these factors will result in failure of the urethra to fuse in the ventral midline, leaving the meatus short of the tip of the glans and the foreskin hooded rather than completely covering the glans.

Most hypospadias is of a relatively minor degree, being glanular or subglanular; both of these are referred to as first-degree hypospadias. Although the urethral plate is present in the glans, there is often a small web of tissue very near the meatus that will deflect the urine stream downward at nearly a right angle to the shaft of the penis. The hooded foreskin produces a phallus that will not be aesthetically acceptable to either the patient or his friends. Although the penis is generally straight and capable of delivering semen into the vagina during sexual intercourse, the angle of the stream and the presence of hooded foreskin are usually sufficient reason to perform surgical repair.

The vast numbers of operative procedures designed to correct hypospadias attest to the fact that no single procedure is entirely satisfactory. Hypospadias that is more severe than glanular or subglanular hypospadias is often accompanied by curvature of the penis, known as a chordee. The chordee may be due to either shortened ventral skin or fibrous tissue between the urethral meatus and the glans penis. The latter probably represents failure of the spongiosum to develop because the urethra did not develop. Determination of the etiology of the curvature is necessary to determine which procedure will be used to repair the hypospadias.

The goal of hypospadias repair is to have a straight penis with a urethra that exits at the tip or very near the tip of the penis. Operative procedures that do not accomplish this goal are not satisfactory. Having tried a number of operative procedures, we have settled on the Duckett procedures as being both capable of producing the desired result and applicable to almost any situation except for the most severe types of perineal hypospadias. Two types of Duckett procedures will be described—the Duckett onlay patch and the Duckett tube graft—both of which use pedicled foreskin with its own blood supply. Studies have not been done to determine the adequacy of this pedicle in supplying blood to the graft, and it may be that it really is not very effective. However, we have performed a large number of these procedures and have found them to be very satisfactory.

With the patient under general anesthesia and using either a dorsal penile block or caudal block with ½% bupivacaine hydrochloride (Marcaine), the foreskin is freed from the glans and cleansed and prepped with povidone-iodine (Betadine). We prefer to do the operative procedure while the patient is still in diapers. The ideal age is between 6 and 12 months, provided the phallus is of reasonable size.

A traction suture is placed just at the end of the urethral plate or the ventral groove of the glans. We use 5-0 Prolene, being careful not to place this traction suture deep to minimize bleeding from the glans. A marking pen is used to outline the circumcision laterally and dorsally around the corona. We usually also mark the dorsal midline of the penile shaft skin to make sure that the dorsal slit, performed later, is as near the midline as possible. The markings on either side of the urethral plate on the ventrum of the penis meet in the midline proximal to the meatus (Fig. 50A). The penile skin just proximal to the meatus is inadequate to support an anastomosis if the markings on the urethral feeding tube can be easily read through the meatal skin. The shaft is then degloved, preserving the blood supply to the skin as much as possible. Hemostasis is secured by judicious use of electrocautery. If, after freeing the shaft skin back as far as the scrotum, there still remains evidence of curvature of the penis, the likelihood of a fibrous chordee is increased. A proximal tourniquet is placed on the penis, using a rubberband placed through a length of red rubber catheter. An artificial erection is then created by injecting sterile saline into the corpora with a 25-gauge butterfly needle (Fig. 50*B1*). If degloving has failed to eliminate the curvature, it will be necessary to divide the urethral plate and construct the urethra using a pedicled tube graft; this procedure is illustrated in column *B* of the figures. If the penis appears straight, the urethra can generally be repaired with an onlay patch urethroplasty; this procedure is illustrated in column *C*. In our experience, the onlay patch is possible in about 90% of patients.

Elimination of the fibrous chordee after division of the urethral plate proximal to the meatus (Fig. 50*B2*) requires dissection of all the white fibrous tissue from the corpora on the ventrum of the penis. This may be a small strip 1 or 2 mm wide, or it may be a wider strip of fibrous tissue of 1 cm or more. Dissection of all of this tissue down to the very bluish fascia over the corpora is necessary. A repeat artificial erection is done to ensure that the penis is as straight as possible. The coronal and glanular urethral plate is left intact. The proximal urethra is trimmed back to good spongiosa tissue for anastomosis to the proximal end of the pedicled tube graft. The length of graft needed can be measured in a number of ways, but using a knife handle ruler seems to be simplest. An extra few millimeters of tube graft are then prepared.

The skin for the graft is dissected free of the shaft skin, protecting the blood supply to both the graft and the shaft skin (Fig. 50*B3*). It is usually not difficult to see the large veins within the shaft skin; the much smaller and nearly invisible arteries run alongside them.

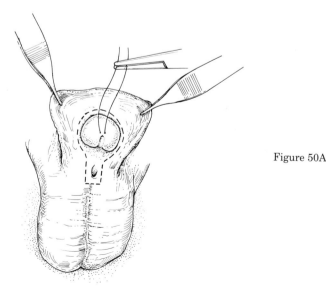

Figure 50A

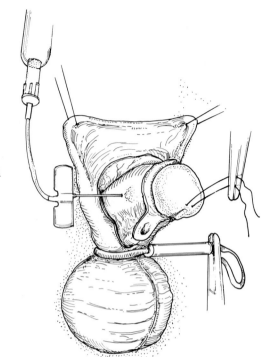

Figure 50B1

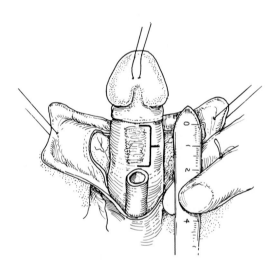

Figure 50B2

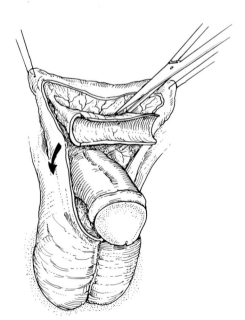

Figure 50B3

The tube graft is constructed using a continuous absorbable suture, for the most part, with interrupted sutures on what will be the distal end of the tube graft so that the graft may be trimmed to length once it is inserted (Fig. 50B4). The tube is constructed over a Silastic catheter; we prefer a 0.04-inch straight Silastic catheter for this purpose. There are two methods of delivering the tube graft to the distal end of the penis. One is by tunneling within the substance of the glans and passing the distal tube up through it (Fig. 50B4, upper inset). Failure to make the tunnel loose enough, in our experience, has resulted in a higher incidence of urethrocutaneous fistula. We prefer to split the glans in the ventral midline and dissect deeply into its substance, creating a bed for the tube graft (Fig. 50B4, upper inset). The proximal end of the tube graft is then sutured to the urethral meatus with a continuous absorbable suture (Fig. 50B4, lower inset). The dorsum of this anastomosis should be attached to the corpora for stability, which seems to reduce the incidence of proximal anastomosis. The suture line of the graft is also placed dorsally against the groove between the two corpora cavernosa.

The catheter used for the construction of the tube graft is then placed into the bladder for postoperative bladder decompression. The meatus is constructed with interrupted absorbable suture (Fig. 50B4, middle inset). If the ventrum of the glans has been split, it is also reconstructed at this time with absorbable interrupted sutures. The interrupted sutures in the distal portion of the tube graft allow it to be tailored to length when creating the meatus so that the graft is not redundant.

A dorsal slit is made on the shaft skin back to where the dorsal skin of the penis is of the correct length. Byar's flaps are then brought around to the ventrum. The deficient ventral skin of the penis is then constructed with either continuous or interrupted absorbable sutures out to where the ventral side of the shaft skin is of reasonable length. The most distal portion of the Byar's flap that contains the knurled bits of hooded foreskin is then trimmed and the circumcision accomplished with continuous or interrupted absorbable sutures (Fig. 50B5).

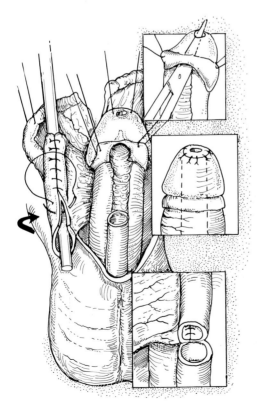

Figure 50B4

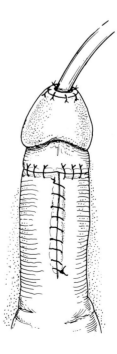

Figure 50–B5

In the patient in whom a pedicle onlay graft is elected, the urethral plate is marked laterally all the way out to the distal end of the glanular groove for later incision (Fig. 50C1). The length of the onlay graft may be similarly measured, providing an extra few millimeters for trimming later.

The foreskin is splayed out with traction sutures so that a rectangle of skin can be developed that is long enough to bridge the gap from the meatus to the tip of the glans, plus a few millimeters (Fig. 50C2).

For the onlay patch urethroplasty, the incisions lateral to the urethral plate (Fig. 50C3) up to the end of the glans are accomplished. Hemostasis in this area is difficult but is aided by the electrocautery. Some surgeons inject dilute epinephrine-lidocaine solution to aid with hemostasis. On occasion, we have placed a tourniquet on the penis because of oozing from this portion of the procedure. A rectangle of foreskin sufficient to provide an onlay patch is cut from the edge of the hooded foreskin.

The onlay patch is sutured to the urethral plate using a long 7-0 Maxon suture. A double-armed suture is placed to fix the proximal end of the onlay patch at the penile meatus (Fig. 50C4). A continuous suture technique is used to approximate the left side of the urethral plate to the onlay patch, all the way to the end of the penis where it is tied. The right side of the urethral meatus and the urethral plate are then joined in a similar fashion so that the graft is performed with a continuous absorbable monofilament suture in a "U" configuration. Before completing the last half of this urethral construction, the same 0.04-inch Silastic catheter is inserted into the bladder for postoperative urinary decompression.

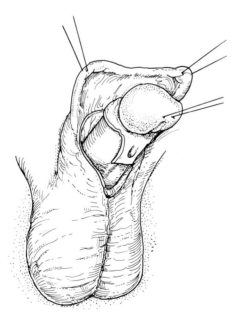

Figure 50C1

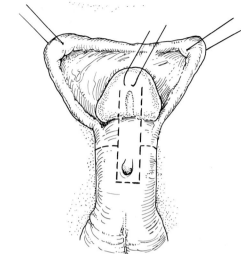

Figure 50C2

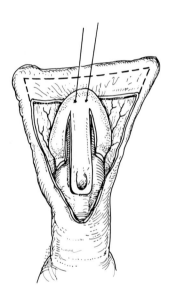

Figure 50C3

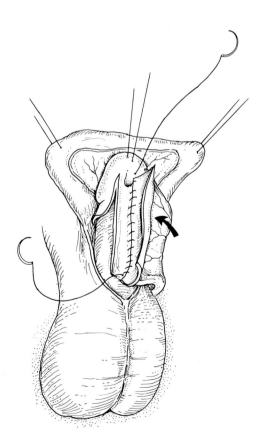

Figure 50C4

Completion of the onlay patch is similar to that for the tube graft except that the ventral side of the glans must be reconstructed (Fig. 50C5). The urethral catheter is transfixed to the glans with a Prolene suture.

Both procedures are then culminated with the application of a molded Silastic sponge dressing (Fig. 50D). This is done by cutting a strip of sterile x-ray film whose width approximately equals the length of the penis. This is formed into a sleeve. Large silk traction sutures are placed in the skin on either side of the base of the penis. The traction sutures are held up along with the penis, which is held by its traction suture. An assistant mixes sponge rubber foam by stirring with its catalyst, and the resulting liquid is poured into the mold formed around the penis. This forms a "muffin"-like dressing, out of which comes the urinary catheter. The two sutures on either side of the penis are tied over the end of the sponge dressing to prevent it from slipping off. The molded dressing prevents suture line stress caused by erection during the critical first 10 postoperative days. Urine drips continuously out of the catheter, which necessitates having the patient in diapers. The open catheter sutured in place appears to be more satisfactory than a Foley catheter. A balloon catheter has a smaller lumen-to-diameter ratio and may become clogged with sediment more easily.

The procedure is done on an outpatient basis. The patients are given a daily dose of urinary antiseptic and two appropriate daily doses of oxybutynin elixir while the catheter remains in place. On approximately the tenth postoperative day, the foam dressing and catheter are removed.

Urethrocutaneous fistula remains a disturbing complication, although experience with the use of the foam dressing indicates that it occurs in less than 5% of patients. Attempts to correct urethrocutaneous fistula should be delayed for at least 6 months until the penile skin softens. Unless the disruption is complete, this can usually be accomplished as an outpatient procedure; it does not require catheter drainage and has a very high likelihood of success.

References

Duckett JW: The island flap technique for hypospadias repair. Urol Clin North Am 8:513–519, 1981.

Duckett JW: Transverse preputial island flap technique for repair of severe hypospadias. Urol Clin North Am 7:423, 1980.

Murphy JP: Hypospadias. In Ashcraft KW, Holder TM, eds: Pediatric Surgery. 2nd ed. Philadelphia, WB Saunders, 1993, pp 694–714.

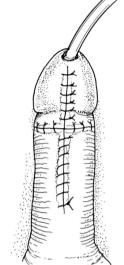

Figure 50C5

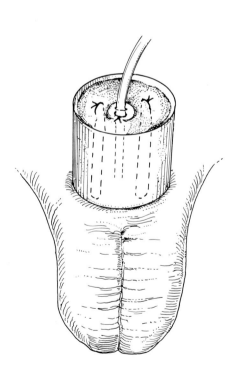

Figure 50D

51

MAGPI
urethroplasty

Most hypospadias is of a relatively minor degree, being glanular or coronal (referred to as first-degree hypospadias). Although the urethral plate is present in the glans, there is often a small web of tissue very near the meatus that will deflect the urine stream downward at nearly a right angle to the shaft of the penis. The hooded foreskin produces a phallus that often looks bent but actually is usually straight. Intercourse and insemination are satisfactory, but the angle of the stream and the presence of hooded foreskin are usually sufficient reasons to perform surgical repair.

The glans is a spade-like, rather than conical, structure. The procedure most commonly used to repair this type of hypospadias is the meatal advancement and glanuloplasty (MAGPI) urethroplasty attributed to Duckett. This can be performed at any age, but we prefer the patient to be between 6 and 12 months old.

The operative procedure is done with the patient under general anesthesia along with a dorsal penile block using ½% bupivacaine (0.3 ml/kg, to a maximum dose of 3 ml). The injection is made just below the symphysis pubis and just above the shaft of the penis, aspirating to ensure that the needle tip is not in the corpora. We place the local anesthetic at a depth of about 2 cm below the pubic skin. It is also possible to perform a caudal block to provide postoperative pain control. This is usually done by the anesthesiologist at the termination of the operative procedure.

Foreskin adhesions are disrupted and the penis cleansed with povidone-iodine (Betadine). A traction suture is placed very shallowly through the skin of the tip of the penis just at the end of the urethral plate. A line is drawn around the corona with a marking pen at the point where the circumcision will be accomplished. An incision is then made all the way around the penis down to the shaft, making sure that the urethra is not entered on the ventral aspect, where it is sometimes thin. This maneuver is best accomplished with a No. 5 or No. 8 feeding tube in the urethra to prevent it from being tented up and inadvertently entered (Fig. 51A).

The shaft of the penis is then degloved almost back to the base, cauterizing vessels as they are encountered. At times a rotational deformity of the penis will be noted, and in these cases it is necessary to continue this dissection more proximally on the penis to derotate it. At this time the web on the urethral plate is incised longitudinally and closed with interrupted absorbable sutures in a transverse fashion. This widens the urethral plate and eliminates the deflecting web that has turned the urinary stream downward (Fig. 51B). The skin on either side of the urethral meatus is undermined to expose the glanular protuberances that will be approximated beneath the urethra as the meatus is moved distally.

The skin of the ventrum of the penis in the midline is then grasped and retracted distally. The ventral skin is approximated so that the meatus is transformed out toward the end of the penis. The glanuloplasty is accomplished by suturing the glanular protuberances together and continuing the approximation of the skin on either side to itself (Fig. 51C). The spade-like glans thus becomes conical. This is likewise best accomplished with a No. 5 or No. 8 feeding tube within the urethra to ensure that luminal diameter is not compromised. The interrupted absorbable sutures may be placed either simply or as mattress sutures. Once the corona has been established on the ventral side of the penis, the shaft skin is once again pulled up. A dorsal slit in the hooded foreskin allows tailoring of the shaft skin to create a straight and aesthetically pleasing penis (Fig. 51D).

We do not leave a stent, nor do we place a molded dressing. Usually petrolatum (Vaseline) or Xeroform gauze is wrapped around the penis along with dry gauze and tape to hold it in place. This provides compression of the penis during the early postoperative hours. The parents are instructed to soak this off in the bathtub later in the day and then to immerse the child in bath water two to three times a day for the next week. The bupivacaine generally

provides good anesthesia for the remainder of the operative day. The following day, acetaminophen (Tylenol) or aspirin is all that is required to provide pain relief.

The results generally are very satisfactory. We have seen only one urethrocutaneous fistula that resulted from dissection to unfold the shaft skin at the meatus.

References

Duckett JW: MAGPI (meatoplasty and glanuloplasty). Urol Clin North Am 8:513–519, 1981.
Murphy JP: Hypospadias. In Ashcraft KW, Holder TM, eds: Pediatric Surgery. 2nd ed. Philadelphia, WB Saunders, 1993, pp 694–714.

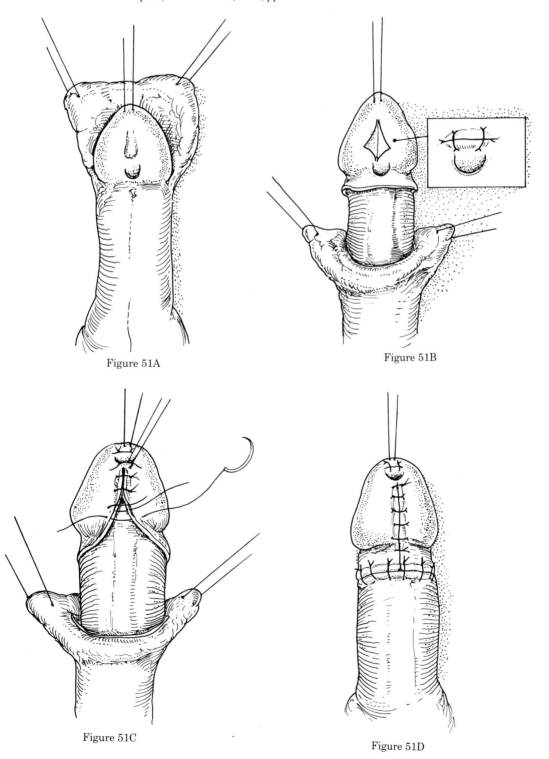

Figure 51A

Figure 51B

Figure 51C

Figure 51D

Adrenogenital syndrome

One of the causes of sexual ambiguity in the newborn is the adrenogenital syndrome, which produces various degrees of masculinization. The defect is in the enzymatic processes by which cholesterol is made into aldosterone, cortisol, and testosterone. The most common enzymatic deficiency is that of 21-hydroxylase, which is necessary in the enzymatic pathway converting progesterone to aldosterone and 17-alpha-hydroxyprogesterone to cortisol. As a consequence, these precursors are shunted to the androgen pathway, and excessive amounts of testosterone are produced. The sensitive tissues of the urogenital sinus respond to the excessive testosterone and its metabolites to form a phallus in the female that would be considered amazingly well developed even in a male.

The patient may appear as having female genitalia with solidly fused labia minora (Fig. 52A1) or as a male with hooded foreskin, chordee, and penoscrotal hypospadias (Fig. 52A2). Rarely will the phallus be complete with a urethra that extends through the glans. Some element of chordee is usually present, and the scrotum is empty (Fig. 52A3).

An enlarged clitoris reminiscent of a glans penis with a urogenital opening at its base is the most common presentation. In the lateral view (Fig. 52B), the confluence of the vagina and urethra may be above the external urethral sphincter or below it (Fig. 52C).

The diagnosis is suspected by inspection and ultimately proved by determination of excessive amounts of 17-hydroxyprogesterone. A buccal smear and chromosome determinations are valuable as well, but a genitogram, accomplished by injection of contrast material into the urogenital sinus, usually reveals the anatomy. The presence of a urogenital sinus, a urethra, a bladder, and a posteriorly located vagina with its cervical indentation provide clear evidence that the anatomy is female. Although not absolutely necessary, early operation can be performed to reduce the size of the phallus and thus eliminate gender ambiguity.

A salt-losing form of adrenogenital syndrome may be present that in times of stress may result in cardiovascular collapse. There may be a history of salt wasting in other siblings or family members. The possibility of this salt-wasting form of adrenogenital syndrome must be kept in mind when dealing with these children.

In a stable patient, clitoris recession may best be accomplished by excising the shaft of the phallus through a hooded incision over the base of the phallus (Fig. 52D).

As in the normal male, sensation to the glans is provided by the dorsal nerve that runs between the bodies of the corpora cavernosa along with the arterial supply to the glans. This blood supply and innervation should be preserved. By lifting and protecting the nerve and vessels, the glans may be freed up and the shaft of the conjoined corpora resected from the level of the corona back to where the corpora bifurcate to attach under the symphysis pubis. The glans is then sutured to the proximal corpora to reduce the size of the phallus, leaving the patient with a clitoris that looks much like a glans penis (Figs. 52E1, 52E2, and 52E3). This method is preferred over simple mobilization of the phallus from the symphysis with recession, because with sexual arousal, the corpora will still engorge, and a very painful bent phallus may interfere with satisfactory sexual activity.

Correction of the urogenital sinus malformation may be done in infancy or delayed until much later. The procedure involves opening the urogenital sinus to separate the urethra from the vagina. If done concomitantly with clitoral resection, the hooded incision over the base of the phallus can be closed and a cutback performed on the urogenital sinus from the base of the phallus.

The posteriorly based skin flap is created when the definitive vaginoplasty is performed (Fig. 52F). This flap may be turned posteriorly while the urethral anatomy is further delineated.

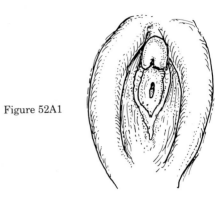

Figure 52A1

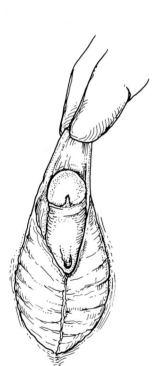

Figure 52A2

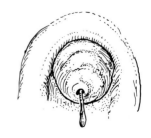

Figure 52A3

Determination of the level of the external sphincter must be made before further cutback. That is best done with a cystoscope, but it is also possible to test this with a nerve stimulator during the open procedure. Endoscopically, the mucosa will appear to be squeezed and will respond to the passage of a cystoscope in the lightly anesthetized patient. If the sphincter (Fig. 52B) surrounds the urethra above the confluence of the vagina and urethra, then a cutback may be accomplished to this point and the urethra need not be elongated to the base of the phallus (Fig. 52G). Further posterior incision will open up the vaginal introitus (Fig. 52H). Labia minora are created by suturing the lateral aspects of the scrotal skin to the lateral walls of the newly opened vagina. The posterior flap then is turned upward to enlarge the introitus (Fig. 52I) and to complete the vaginoplasty.

When the external urinary sphincter (Fig. 52J) is determined to be below the confluence of the vagina and urethra, then a different approach must be taken. A small Foley catheter or Fogarty catheter is inserted through the urethra, and dissection is carried up along the ventral side of the urethra to the sphincter and above. The inflated balloon in the vagina allows easy identification of that structure so that it may be opened above the external sphincter. The vagina is then detached from the presphincteric urethra and prepared for the introital construction (Fig. 52K).

The urethra above the sphincter is closed with interrupted sutures, being careful not to constrict the lumen. The short vagina is opened in a fish-mouth fashion. The urethra beyond the sphincter is then sewn to the anterior portion of the open vagina. The posterior portion is attached to the posteriorly based flap (Fig. 52L) and the labia are then reconstructed out of the rugated, fused labioscrotal skin flaps on either side (Fig. 52M). Thus a complex closure is accomplished; this is shown in a cutaway drawing in Figure 52N.

The most common problem after an operation of this type is stenosis of the vaginal introitus. Therefore, the vaginoplasty portion is sometimes delayed until near puberty. A stricture may result in difficult or impossible intercourse, requiring revision of the vaginoplasty at the time of impending sexual activity.

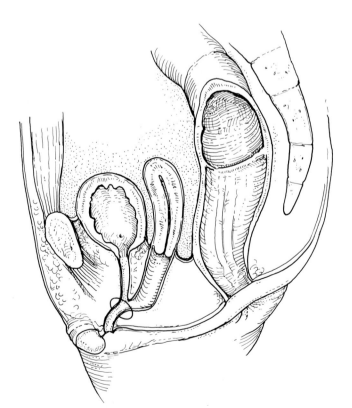

Figure 52B

Reference

Donahoe PK, Powell DM: Treatment of intersex abnormalities. In Ashcraft KW, Holder TM, eds: Pediatric Surgery. 2nd ed. Philadelphia, WB Saunders, 1993, pp 740–765.

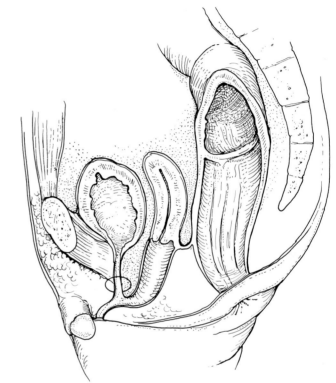

Figure 52C

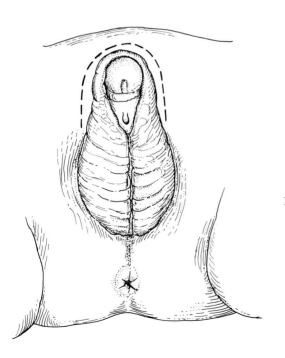

Figure 52D

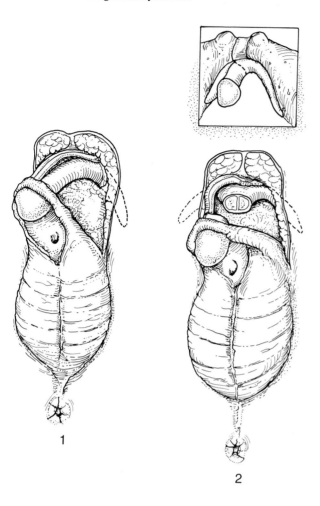

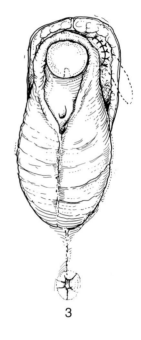

1

2

3

Figure 52E

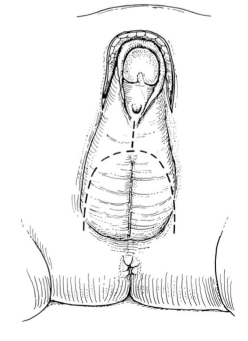

Figure 52F

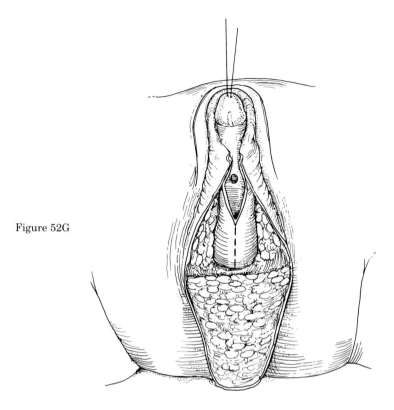

Figure 52G

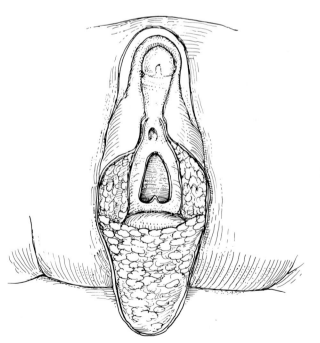

Figure 52H

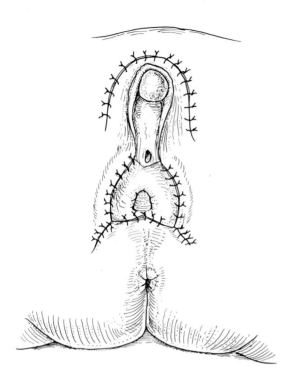

Figure 52I

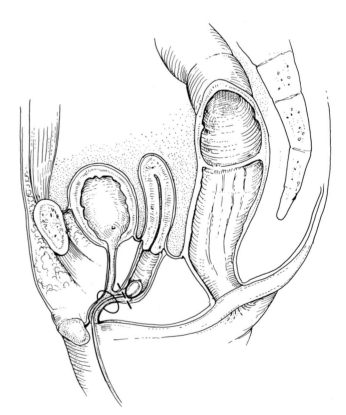

Figure 52J

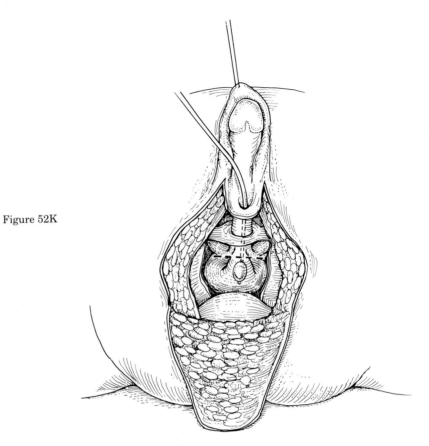

Figure 52K

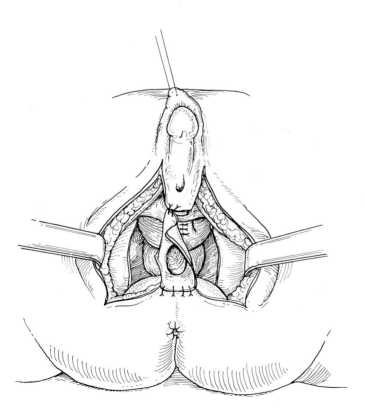

Figure 52L

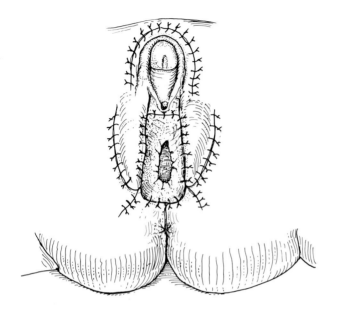

Figure 52M

Figure 52N

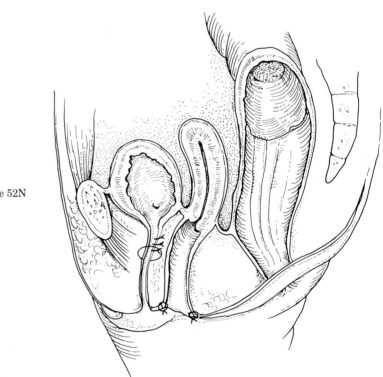

INDEX

Note: Italicized numbers indicate illustrations.

A

Abscess, perirectal, 230
Acetaminophen, 286, 303
n-Acetylcysteine, 150, 152
Achalasia, 75–75, *77–78*
Adrenogenital syndrome, 305–308, *307–314*
Aganglionosis, 174, 210–212
Airway obstruction, 14, 18
Aldosterone, 306
Ammonia intoxication, 134
Anastomosis
  circumferential, 210, *211*
  for colon interposition, 54, *53, 55*
  for gastric tube, 58–60, *59*
  for intestinal atresia, 142–144
  for meconium ileus, 150
  for enterocolitis, 156
  for tracheoesophageal fistula, 40, 42, *43*
  ileoanal, 234
  side-to-side, 212, *213*
Anesthesia, vascular access for, 22, *23*
Anorectoplasty, 186, 240
Antral duplication, *166*
Anus, imperforate, 174, 186, 187
Aorta, coarctation of, 156
Arteries. *See named vessels, e.g.,* Testicular artery.
Aspirin, 286, 303
Atresia
  biliary, 104–109, 134
  duodenal, 92, *92*
  esophageal, 37–42, *38–41, 43*
  intestinal, 139–146, *141–147,* 150, 182

B

Barrett's esophagus. *See* Esophagus, Barrett's.
"Bell clapper" deformity, 286
Benson pyloric spreader, 87, *87*
Biliary atresia, 104–109, 134
Blind loop syndrome, 150
Bowel
  exteriorization of, 156
  gangrene of, 100, 156
  inflammation of, 182
Bowel *(Continued)*
  obstruction of, 98, 150, 280
Branchial cleft sinus, 11–12, *12*
Bupivacaine hydrochloride, 254, 259, 292, 302
Byar's flap, 295

C

Caroli's disease, 113–114
Chest tube, 26, 42, *43*, 64
"Chimney" procedure, 150, *152*
"Chinese" technique, 200, 206
Choledochal cyst, 111–116, *112–115*
Choledochojejunostomy, 104, 109
Cholesterol, 306
Cholestyramine ointment, 194
Chordee, 292, 306
"Christmas tree" deformity, 140, *141, 146, 147,* 156
Clatworthy procedure, 134
Cloaca, 239–246, *240–247*
Colectomy, 234
Colitis, ulcerative, 234
Collodion, 8
Colon, interposition of, 49–56, *51, 53, 55–56*
Colostomy, 173–176, *175, 177*
  complications of, 176
  divided, 174–176, *175, 177*
  leveling, 176, *177*
Cryptotomy, 230
Cystic fibrosis, 134
  meconium ileus and, 150, 152
  rectal prolapse and, 216
Cystoscopy, 308
Cyst(s)
  choledochal, 111–116, *112–115*
  dermoid, 6
  duplication, 166, *167*
  preauricular, 7–8, *9*
  thyroglossal, 13–14, *15*

D

Dartos pouch, 270–272, *274–275*
Decompression
  ileostomy, 150, *152*

Decompression *(Continued)*
    nasogastric, 72
    portal, 128
Dermoids, 5–6, *6*
Diatrizoate meglumine, 150
Dihydrotestosterone, 292
Down syndrome, duodenal atresia and, 95
Drapanas shunt, 134, *134*
Duckett urethroplasty, 291–298, *293–297, 299*
Duct
    thyroglossal, 13–14, *15*
    Wirsung, 122, *122*
Duhamel procedure, 200, 205–212, *207–213*
Duodenal atresia, 92, 95, *93*
Duodenal obstruction, 91–96, *92–95*

E

Ear, preauricular sinus of, 7–8, *9*
Ectopic testes, *268*
Empyema, thoracotomy for, 25–26, *27*
Endorectal pull-through, 233–234, *235–237*
Enterocolitis, necrotizing. *See* Necrotizing
    enterocolitis (NEC).
Epididymitis, 286–288
Epinephrine, 296
Esophageal atresia, 37–42, *38–41, 43*
Esophagus
    Barrett's, 68
    colon interposition for, 49–56, *51, 53, 55–56*
    gastric tube for, 57–60, *58–59*
    varices in, 128
Eyebrow, dermoid on, 6

F

Familial polyposis, 234
Fecaloma, 212
Femoral vein, vascular access by, 22, *23*
Fertility
    testicular torsion and, 288
    undescended testis and, 270
Fistula
    from cloaca repair, 246
    rectal fourchette, 186, *187*, 190, *191*
    rectoperitoneal, 186, *187*, 190, *191*
    tracheoesophageal, *38*
    urethrocutaneous, 298, 303
Fistula-in-ano, 229–230, *230–231*
Fowler-Stephens procedure, 270
Fundoplication, 67–72, *69–71, 73*
    complications of, 72
    for achalasia, 76, *77–78*

G

Ganglioneuroma, 46
Gangrene, 100
Gas bloat syndrome, 72
Gastric tube, 57–60, *58–59*
Gastroesophageal (GE) reflux
    from gastric tube, 60
    medication for, 68
    surgery for, 68
Gastrografin. *See* Diatrizoate meglumine.
Gastrojejunostomy, 124
Gastroschisis, 156, 179–182, *180–282*
Gastrostomy, 60
    Stamm, 79–82, *81–83*
GE reflux. *See* Gastroesophageal (GE) reflux.
Gender ambiguity, 306
Gonadotropin-releasing hormone, 268

Gore-Tex, 62
Granuloplasty, 302

H

Haemophilus influenzae, 26
Hand vein, vascular access by, 22, *23*
Hartmann's pouch, 176, *177*, 200, 206–210,
    234
Heart disease, congenital, cyanotic, 156
Heller myotomy, 76, *77–78*
Hematoma
    airway obstruction from, 14
    sinus repair and, 12
Hepatitis, neonatal, 105
Hernia
    diaphragmatic, 61–64, *62–65*
    hiatal, 68
    inguinal, 249–261, *250–261*
    recurrence of, 261
    umbilical, 263–264, *265*
Hilum, adenopathy of, 46
Hirschsprung's disease, 174, 176, 200, 206
Histoplasmosis, 46
Hydrocele, 250
17-Hydroxyprogesterone, 306
Hyperinsulinism, 122
Hypersplenism, 134
Hypertension
    portal, 128
    pulmonary, 64
Hypospadias, 292–298, *293–297, 299,* 302–
    303, *303*

I

Ileal reservoir, 234, *237*
Ileoanal anastomosis, 234
Ileostomy
    decompression, 150, *152*
    Mikulicz, 150
    protective, 234
Ileus, meconium, 149–152, *151–153*
Incisions, 1–2, *2–3*
Inguinal hernia, 249–261, *250–261*
Intestinal atresia, 139–146, *141–147,* 150, 182
Intestinal duplication, 165–166, *166–167*
Intestinal obstruction, 98, 150, 280
Intussusception, 161–162, *163–164*
    rectal prolapse vs., 216, 218

J

"J"-shaped reservoir, 234, *237*

K

Kasai procedure, 103–110, *104–109*
Kidney
    agenesis of, 240
    tumor of, 278

L

Ladd's bands, 98, 100
Langhorn, lines of, 2
Laryngeal lesion, 18
Leveling colostomy, 176, *177*
Lidocaine, 296

Lipoma, 250
Liver transplantation, 104, 113, 128
Loop colostomy, 174, *175*
Lymphoma, 46

M

MAGPI urethroplasty, 301–303, *303*
Malrotation, 97–100, *98–101,* 182
Marasmus, 68
Marcaine. *See* Bupivacaine hydrochloride.
Martin procedure, 210
Masculinization, 306
Meckel's diverticulum, 169–170, *171*
Meconium ileus, 149–152, *151–153*
Mediastinal lesions, 45–46, *47–48*
Mesocaval shunt, 133–134, *135–137*
Mikulicz ileostomy, 150
Milk of magnesia, 194
Mini-Pena procedure, 185–186, *187. See also*
    Pena procedure.
Mucomyst. *See* n-Acetylcysteine.
Myasthenia gravis, 46
Myotomy. *See also* Pylomyotomy.
    Heller, 76, *77–78*
Myringotomy, 250

N

Nasogastric decompression, 72
NEC. *See* Necrotizing enterocolitis (NEC).
Neck dermoid, 6
Necrotizing enterocolitis (NEC), 146, 155–158,
    157, 159
Nephrectomy, 280
Neuroblastoma, 46
Nissen fundoplication, 68–72, *73*
    complications of, 72
Nutrition, parenteral. *See* Total parenteral
    nutrition.

O

Omphalocele, 179–182, *180–282*
Orchiopexy, 267–272, *268–275*
Otitis, 250
Ovary, reduction of, 252
Oxybutynin, 298

P

Pain control, 254, 286, 303. *See also* Patient-
    controlled analgesia.
Pancreas, annular, 94
Pancreatectomy, 121–126, *122–123, 125*
    complications of, 124
    distal, 123, *123*
    subtotal, 124, *123, 125*
Parenteral nutrition. *See* Total parenteral
    nutrition.
Patent ductus arteriosus, 156
Patient-controlled analgesia (PCA), 34. *See*
    also Pain control.
Pectus carinatum, 34
Pectus excavatum, 29–35, *30–33, 35*
Pena procedure, 189–197, *190–193, 195–196.*
    See also Mini-Penaprocedure.
Peptic ulceration, 170
Perichondrium, reefing of, 33, *33*
Perirectal abscess, 230
Peritonitis, 150, 156

Peyer's patch, 162
Pneumonitis, 38, 68
Polyposis, familial, 234
Portal decompression, 128
Portocaval shunt, 133–134, *135–137*
Portoenterostomy, 103–110, *104–109*
Posterior sagittal anorectoplasty. *See* Pena
    procedure.
Preauricular cyst, 7–8, *9*
Presacral teratoma, 225–226, *227–228*
Prolapse
    rectal, 215–218, *216–218*
    stomal, 176
Pull-through, endorectal, 233–234, *235–237*
Pulmonary hypoplasia, 64
Pylomyotomy, 85–89, *86–88. See also*
    Myotomy.

R

Rectal fourchette fistula, 186, *187*
Rectal prolapse, 215–218, *216–218*
Rectoperitoneal fistula, 186, *187,* 191,*191*
5-alpha-Reductase, 292
Reefing, of perichondrium, 33, *33*
Reflux, gastroesophageal
    from gastric tube, 60
    medication for, 68
    surgery for, 68
Reservoir, ileal, 234, *237*
Rotational deformity, 302
Roux-en-Y jejunostomy, 104, 109, 114

S

Sacrococcygeal teratoma, 219–222, *220–223*
Saphenous vein, vascular access by, 22, *23*
Scarring, 2
Sclerotherapy, 128
Scrotum, acute, 285–288, *286–289*
Shiley tube, 18
Short gut syndrome, 146, 158, 182
Shunt
    decompression, 128
    Drapanas, 134, *134*
    mesocaval, 133–134, *135–137*
    portocaval, 133–134, *135–137*
    splenorenal, 127–128, *129–131*
SIDS. *See* Sudden infant death syndrome
    (SIDS).
"Silk glove" sign, 250
Sinus
    branchial cleft, 11–12, *12*
    preauricular, 7–8, *9*
Skin cyst, 6
Soave pull-through, 199–200, *201–203*
Splenectomy, 117–118, *118–119*
    after portocaval shunt, 134
Splenorenal shunt, 127–128, *129–131*
"S"-shaped reservoir, 234, *237*
Stamm gastrostomy, 79–82, *81–83*
Staphylococcal infection, 26
Steroid therapy, 46
Stoma, prolapse of, 176
Sudden infant death syndrome (SIDS), 68

T

Technetium 99m scan, 170
Teratoma
    mediastinal, 46
    presacral, 225–226, *227–228*

Teratoma *(Continued)*
  sacrococcygeal, 219–222, *220–223*
Testicular artery, 270
Testis(es)
  dysplastic, 270
  ectopic, *268*
  retractile, 268
  torsion of, *286,* 286–288
  undescended, 263–264, *265*
    bilateral, 272
    fertility and, 270
Testosterone, 292, 306
Thal fundoplication, 68–70, *69–71*
  complications of, 72
  for achalasia, 76, *77–78*
Thoracentesis, 26
Thoracoscopy, 26
Thoracotomy, for empyema, 25–26, *27*
Thrombus, tumor, 280
Thymectomy, 46
Thyroglossal cyst, 13–14, *15*
Torsion, testicular, *286,* 286–288
Total parenteral nutrition
  after intestinal atresia, 146
  for duodenal obstruction, 95
  vascular access for, 22–24, *23*
Tracheoesophageal fistula, *38*
Tracheostomy, 17–18, *19*
Tylenol. *See* Acetaminophen.

U

UDTs. *See* Undescended testes (UDTs).
Ulceration, peptic, 170
Ulcerative colitis, 234
Umbilical hernia, 263–264, *265*
Undescended testes (UDTs), 263–264, *265*
  bilateral, 272

Undescended testes (UDTs) *(Continued)*
  misdiagnosis of, 268
Urethrocutaneous fistula, 298, 303
Urethroplasty
  Duckett, 291–298, *293–297, 299*
  MAGPI, 301–303, *303*

V

VACTERL. *See* Vertebral, anal, cardiac,
    tracheal, esophageal,renal, and limb
    (VACTERL) defects.
Vagina
  bifid, 240
  fistula in, 190, 192, 194, *191*
  septate, 240
Vagus nerve, 38
Varices, esophageal, 128
Vascular access, 21–24, *23*
Veins. *See specific vessels, e.g.,* Saphenous
    vein.
Vertebral, anal, cardiac, tracheal, esophageal,
    renal, and limb
    (VACTERL) defects, 38
Vesicoureteric reflux, 240
Volvulus, 100, 150

W

Whipple procedure, 124
Wilms' tumor, 277–280, *278–284*
Wirsung, duct of, 122, *123*

X

Xiphoid, removal of, 32, *32*

ISBN 0-7216-3720-5

90038